EAT THIS NOT THAT!

Thousands of Simple Food Swaps That Can Save You 10, 20, 30 Pounds—or More!

BY DAVID ZINCZENKO

Editor-in-Chief of **Men'sHealth**

WITH MATT GOULDING

RODALE

Notice

Mention of specific companies, organizations, or authorities in this book does not imply endorsement by the publisher, nor does mention of specific companies, organizations, or authorities imply that they endorse this book.

The brand-name products mentioned in this book are trademarks or registered trademarks of their respective companies. This book should not be regarded as a substitute for professional medical treatment, and neither the author, publisher, manufacturers, or distributors can accept legal responsibility for any problem arising out of the use of or experimentation with the methods described.

Nutrition information for all brand-name products mentioned in this book was provided by their companies or on official nutrition labels. Applebee's International, Inc., Outback Steakhouse (OSI Restaurant Partners, LLC), Red Lobster (Darden Restaurants, Inc.), Olive Garden (Darden Restaurants, Inc.), and Sbarro do not provide complete nutrition information to the public; the estimates for their products were obtained from CalorieKing.com, an independent nutrition information and communication service that is owned and operated by Family Health Publications Pty Ltd.

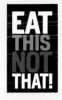
EAT
THIS
NOT
THAT!

DEDICATION

To fast food and chain restaurants like Burger King, Chili's, and Panera, among others, that have made it a priority to provide comprehensive nutritional information for their products: Your transparency has gone a long way in helping us arm consumers with a road map for making smart choices when eating out.

Sadly, many of the largest chain restaurants in this country continue to obscure, disguise, or completely conceal the calorie, fat, and sodium counts for their food. This type of nutritional negligence, one that denies consumers even the most basic understanding of what they're putting in their bodies, poses a major health threat to this country. To those restaurants, including Applebee's, Olive Garden, Outback, Red Lobster, TGI Friday's, and others, we hope this book plays some part, small or large, in compelling you to provide what every diner in America deserves: full disclosure.

In the much-talked-about obesity crisis in America, chain restaurants are a major player. From New York to California, the restaurant industry continues to dump millions of dollars into lobbying against government initiatives that would force them to provide nutritional information for their consumers. They claim that the answer to the obesity crisis is education. We couldn't agree more. That's why we're publishing this book.

ACKNOWLEDGMENTS

This book is the product of thousands of meals, hundreds of menu experiments, and the collective smarts, dedication, and raw talent of dozens of individuals. Our undying thanks to all of you who have inspired this project in any way. In particular:

Steve Murphy, who captains the ship called Rodale, Inc. with grace, courage, and remarkable vision. Thanks for continuing to make this the best publishing company on the planet.

The Rodale family, whose dedication to improving the lives and well-being of their readers is apparent in every book and magazine they put their name on.

George Karabotsos, whose vision has turned a jumble of words and numbers into something that's impossible to put down.

Stephen Perrine, with whom we've conferred over many a fast-food lunch, and who never met an exclamation mark he didn't like.

Paul Reader, whose unyielding dedication on the part of *Men's Health* and Rodale have helped spread the word about health, fitness, and nutrition to millions of Americans.

Lauren Murrow, whose tireless efforts and editorial savvy are the glue that holds these pages together.

To the Rodale book team: Liz Perl, Bob Anderson, Chris Krogermeier, Kevin Smith, Marina Padakis, Tara Long, Keith Biery, and Anita Patterson. Your extraordinary sacrifices of time and sanity brought this project to reality in record time.

The entire *Men's Health* editorial staff: a smarter, more inspiring group of writers, editors, researchers, designers, and photo directors does not exist, in the magazine world or beyond.

Special thanks to: Adam Campbell, Ben Hewitt, Mark Michaelson, Peter Moore, David Schipper, Kyle Western, and Laura White.

And to the people who matter most to us in this world: Families, friends, and our lovely partners, Melissa and Lauren.

Sorry for all the talk about calorie counts.

—Dave and Matt

CONTENTS

A Weight Loss Coach in Your Pocket

I don't want you to read this book.

I don't want you to read this book because I want you to do something else: I want you to USE it.

Use it when you're out with friends. Use it when you're shopping for your family. Use it when you're idling in the drive-thru, waiting to talk to a clown. Use it to make smart, healthy, fat-busting food choices no matter where you are. Use it to strip away belly fat, build lean, firm muscle, and *look and feel fitter, healthier, and happier than you have in years.*

See, this isn't a traditional diet book. Diet books are great when you're sitting at home and reading. But how do they help you out in the real world, where an impatient server or a kid in a paper hat is waiting for your decision? Besides, I bet you have better things to do than to sit inside reading diet books. Instead, you'd rather be out in the world enjoying yourself—having fun with office mates, sharing good times with family—and knowing that you're making the right food choices every time. It's simple: Just use **EAT THIS, NOT THAT!** as your sourcebook, and you can live life to the fullest and still lose weight and build the body you want.

Smart weight loss isn't about starving yourself, or eating only grapefruit and tofu, or running everything you eat through a juicer (which really ruins the pizza experience, by the way). The smart path to weight loss is about smart choices—choices you make every day.

With **EAT THIS, NOT THAT!**, those choices just got easier.

As the editor-in-chief of *Men's Health* magazine, it's my job to scour the studies, interview the experts, test out the trends, and compile the newest, smartest, most authoritative information on weight loss available. I even created my own diet franchise—The Abs Diet—which has sold more than one million copies, much of it by word-of-mouth. And it works! Tens of thousands of men and women have lost weight and rediscovered the firm, rippled abdominal muscles of their youth—and gained control of their waistlines, their health, and their lives.

So why *EAT THIS, NOT THAT!?*

It's simple. No matter how successful The Abs Diet has been, it shares with all other diets one single dilemma: A diet only works if you have control over what, how, and when you're eating. And as you well know, most of the time, you don't have control.

Sure, you can cook your own dinner. You can brown-bag your own lunch. You can spoon yourself some yogurt in the morning and eat a healthy snack before bedtime. (And yes, there ARE healthy and delicious snacks to eat before bedtime.) But you can't control what's offered at the office cafeteria (unless you own the company), or what's being served at Mom's house for Thanksgiving (unless you're Mom). And you can't stand in the kitchen at Olive Garden or Mickey D's and tell the chef to go easier on the vegetable oil, either.

Consider this:

TWO-THIRDS OF U.S. ADULTS ARE NOW OVERWEIGHT, and the obesity rate has increased 50 percent since 1960. Is it because we all just turned into junk food junkies? No: It's because restaurants and packaged food marketers are loading our meals with empty calories, and there's nothing we can do about it—until now, that is!

THE FOOD INDUSTRY SPENDS $30 BILLION A YEAR ON ADVERTISING— 70 percent of it pitching convenience foods, candy, soda, and desserts. Even the teens working behind the counter are coached to get you to upsize your meal. (And for an average 17 percent more money, you get yourself 55 percent more calories! A bargain—if you consider flab a good investment.)

EVEN THE EXPERTS ARE CONFUSED. In a Cornell University study, 85 grad students and nutrition science professors served themselves ice cream. One group underestimated their own serving size—and caloric intake—by 40 percent!

But with *EAT THIS, NOT THAT!*, you're the expert. You're the expert in the frozen food aisle. You're the expert at the deli counter. You're even the expert at the sushi restaurant. You control your food universe because, unlike every other customer, you'll know the smart choices to make—instantly!

Just think about what this means:

YOU'LL LOSE WEIGHT.
EAT THIS, NOT THAT is crafted to specifically target belly fat—by filling you with smart, healthy choices that rev up your resting metabolism and help you burn away flab all day, every day, even while you sleep!

YOU'LL RESHAPE YOUR BODY.
Most diet plans force you to cut, cut, cut calories until you're practically starving. And what do you get? Sure, you lose fat, but you also lose muscle. And muscle is crucial to keeping your metabolism revving and giving you the lean, firm shape you crave. So as soon as you go off your starvation diet, your body is primed to gain weight back more easily than before. But with *EAT THIS, NOT THAT!*, you'll never go hungry. You'll eat in the same places at the same times, but you'll eat smarter. And that means you'll be able to hold on to—and even build—firm, lean muscle while shedding useless, flabby pounds.

YOU'LL GAIN GREATER HEALTH.
The number-one principle of *EAT THIS, NOT THAT!* is to cut empty calories and add in nutrition—more bang for your caloric buck with every bite. And by carving away belly flab, you'll cut your risk of heart disease, diabetes, stroke,

and even cancer. (A University of Alabama-Birmingham study, for example, found that the amount of belly flab you carry is the single best predictor of heart disease—more so than blood pressure, cholesterol, or family history.)

YOU'LL EVEN GAIN RESPECT.
Not just the respect of those who admire your body—because let's face it, staying lean is something successful people do—but the respect of coworkers and bosses, too. Don't believe me? Consider this: An NYU study found that people packing on an extra 40 pounds make 20 percent less than their slimmer colleagues.

Those are some hefty promises, but *EAT THIS, NOT THAT!* has the insider info to deliver.

Think about it: Do you really know what's in the food you're ordering at the sports bar, the fast food restaurant, the local diner, or the all-you-can-eat buffet? Not unless you've worked in the kitchen yourself. Do you really know if that burger is 250 calories, or 500 calories, or 1,000 calories? No. (And you'll be shocked and amazed when you discover the truth!)

Well, now you'll know. And you'll be able to make smart choices wherever you go, whenever you go. Losing weight and feeling fit and healthy has never been so easy. And there's a reason for that:

EAT THIS, NOT THAT! **is jam-packed with SECRETS THE RESTAURANT INDUSTRY DOESN'T WANT YOU TO KNOW! For example:**

BURGER KING doesn't want you to know that a BK Big Fish® Sandwich and fries have a whopping 1,000 calories—nearly half your daily caloric intake! (Fish is usually healthy, but not this kind. Find out why on page 39.)

PIZZA HUT doesn't want you to know that a standard pizza in Italy contains 500 to 800 calories, but the same meal at Pizza Hut can top 2,100 calories! (You'd need to ride a stationary bike for more than three hours to burn off this mistake. Instead, eat all the pizza you want by making smart choices—I've outlined them on page 106.)

PANERA doesn't want you to know that their Sierra Turkey sandwich packs 40 grams of fat! (The real criminal is the bread it's served on—check out page 103 for details.)

MACARONI GRILL doesn't want you to know that a single serving of their Grilled Salmon Teriyaki has more than three times your daily allowance of sodium! (Cut your risk of high blood pressure by making smart choices at the same restaurant. You'll find them on page 117.)

APPLEBEE'S, OLIVE GARDEN, OUTBACK, and **RED LOBSTER** don't want you to know that they don't provide full nutritional information for their products. We had a hunch these titans of the restaurant industry were hiding something, so we teamed up with the nutritional analysis website CalorieKing.com to uncover the numbers for these last few stubborn holdouts, and what we found was astounding: A plate of Chicken Marsala at Olive Garden has 1,315 calories and 86 grams of fat; a *salad* at Applebee's (their Grilled Steak Caesar) has more than an entire day's worth of fat entangled in its leaves; and Outback's Aussie Cheese Fries, at 2,900 calories, is the single worst food in America. (Start your own investigation on page 6.)

No, the restaurant and packaged-food industries don't want you to know any of this. They want you to go right ahead and keep ordering their food blindly, trying to eat healthy but never really knowing what's in that not-so-happy meal in front of you, and wondering why the weight never seems to come off.

The funny thing is, if you only knew the insider information, you could eat at any of your favorite restaurants—or chow down on everything from the company vending machine to your kids' Halloween buckets—and know that every decision you made was smart, healthy, and the best possible choice for you. For example, did you know:

AT KRISPY KREME, all you need to do is order the Very Berry Chiller instead of the Mocha Dream Chiller, and you'll save 500 calories? (Do that once a week and you'll drop more than 7 pounds this year—without trying!)

AT CHIPOTLE, you can cut 498 calories out of your Chicken Burrito just by ordering it as a bowl (without the tortilla) and asking them to hold the rice. (Same great taste, but with 94 fewer carb grams!)

AT COLD STONE CREAMERY, you can save 40 calories and 2 grams of fat by choosing shaved chocolate, not chocolate chips, as your topping. (Sure, you're indulging—but why not indulge smartly?)

AT McDONALD'S, an Egg McMuffin® is actually a healthy choice, with just 300 calories. (The Hotcakes pack more than double that amount!)

AT CHICK-FIL-A, not a single sandwich tops 500 calories. (When it comes to fast food, this might be the healthiest no-brainer around.)

IN THE PRODUCE AISLE, you'll get twice the vitamin C—and nine times as much vitamin A—by simply picking red bell peppers over green ones. (Who said eating healthy was difficult?)

And that's why **EAT THIS, NOT THAT!** is going to change everything. It's time to level the playing field. We're all tired of sneaky calories adding to our waistlines, and having to starve ourselves or spend hours on the treadmill trying to burn off the damage. Now—for the first time—you're in charge!

For more great food swaps, nutritional secrets, quick and simple recipes, weight-loss tactics, and the latest breaking news on staying lean and feeling great, go to **menshealth.com/eatthis**

Cheeseburger

Eat This
McDonald's Big Mac®
540 calories 29 g fat

Not That!
Burger King Whopper® with Cheese
760 calories 47 g fat

Save 220 calories and 18 grams of fat!

Pizza

Eat This
2 slices Domino's large cheese pizza with hand-tossed crust
580 calories 18 g fat

Not That!
2 slices Pizza Hut large cheese pizza with hand-tossed crust
680 calories 28 g fat

Save 100 calories and 10 grams of fat!

Turkey Sandwich

Eat This
Subway 6-inch Turkey Sub with Cheese
330 calories 8.5 g fat

Not That!
Panera Sierra Turkey
840 calories 40 g fat

Save 510 calories and 31.5 grams of fat!

Fish Sandwich

Eat This
McDonald's Filet-O-Fish®
380 calories 18 g fat

Not That!
Burger King Big Fish® Sandwich
640 calories 32 g fat

Save 260 calories and 14 grams of fat!

Burrito

Eat This
Taco Bell Regular Style Steak Burrito Supreme
390 calories 14 g fat

Not That!
Chipotle Steak Burrito
1,126 calories 45 g fat

Save 736 calories and 31 grams of fat!

Caesar Salad

Eat This
Panera Chicken Caesar Salad
560 calories   34 g fat

Not That!
Chili's Chicken Caesar Salad
1,010 calories   76 g fat

Save 450 calories and 42 grams of fat!

Breakfast Sandwich

Eat This
McDonald's Egg McMuffin®
300 calories   12 g fat

Not That!
Starbucks Classic Sausage, Egg, & Aged Cheddar Breakfast Sandwich
460 calories   25 g fat

Save 160 calories and 13 grams of fat!

Cinnamon Roll

Eat This
Au Bon Pain Cinnamon Roll
350 calories   12 g fat

Not That!
Cinnabon® Classic Cinnamon Roll
813 calories   32 g fat

Save 463 calories and 20 grams of fat!

Donuts

Eat This
Krispy Kreme Original Glazed Doughnut
200 calories   12 g fat

Not That!
Dunkin' Donuts Glazed Cake Donut
33U calories   18 g fat

Save 130 calories and 6 grams of fat!

Banana Split

Eat This
Dairy Queen Classic Banana Split
530 calories   12 g fat

Not That!
Baskin-Robbins Banana Split
1,030 calories   39 g fat

Save 500 calories and 27 grams of fat!

PHOTO CREDITS

Craig Cutler: pp. 6, 7, 13

Nicholas Eveleigh, photographer; **Karen Temple**, food stylist: pp. 226-227

John Hamel, photographer; **Melissa Reiss**, food stylist: pp. 16, 17, 18, 19, 20, 21, 22, 23, 24, 25, 28, 29, 32, 33, 34, 35, 36, 37, 38, 39, 44, 45, 46, 47, 52, 53, 56, 57, 58, 59, 60, 62, 63, 70, 71, 82, 83, 88, 89, 92, 93, 94, 95, 98, 99, 102, 103, 104, 105, 106, 107, 112, 113, 114, 115, 118, 119, 128, 129, 130, 131, 132, 133, 136, 137, 170, 171, 172, 173, 174, 175, 176, 177, 178, 179, 180, 181, 182, 183, 184, 185, 186, 187, 188, 189, 190, 191, 192, 193

Jeff Harris, photographer; **Susan Sugarman**, food stylist: Cover photos, pp. 274-275

Michael Heiko: pp. 262-263

Laura Johansen, photographer; **Tracy Harlor**, food stylist: pp. 172-173

Michael LoBiondo; **John Hartley**, food stylist: pp. 50, 51, 64, 65, 68, 69, 72 , 73, 80, 81, 84, 85, 86, 87, 91, 100, 101, 108, 109, 116, 117, 120, 121, 122, 123, 134, 135

Thomas MacDonald/Rodale Images: pp. 196, 197, 198, 199, 200, 201, 202, 203, 204, 205, 206, 207, 208, 209, 210, 211, 212, 213, 214, 215, 216, 217, 218, 219, 220, 221, 222, 223, 224, 225, 228, 229, 230, 231, 232, 233, 234, 235, 236, 237, 238, 239, 240, 241, 242, 243, 244, 245, 246, 247, 248, 249, 250, 251, 252, 253

Mitch Mandel/Rodale Images; **Melissa Reiss**, food stylist: pp. 256, 257, 258, 259, 260, 261, 264, 265, 266, 267, 270, 271

Orly Katz: pp. 26, 27, 30, 31, 40, 41, 42, 43, 48, 49, 54, 55, 66, 67, 74, 75, 76, 77, 78, 79, 90, 96, 97, 110, 111, 124, 125, 126, 127

Melissa Punch: pp. 140, 141, 142, 143, 144, 145, 146, 147, 148, 149, 150, 151, 152, 153, 154, 155, 156, 157, 158, 159, 160, 161, 162, 163, 164, 165

James Worrell: pp. 166-167

Portions of 8 Foods You Should Eat Every Day, by **Ben Hewitt**, appeared in *Best Life*.

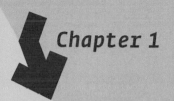

Chapter 1

8 FOODS YOU SHOULD EAT EVERY DAY
PLUS: 20 to avoid at all costs

8 Foods You Should Eat Every Day

It sometimes seems as if the internal politics of the Middle East are easier to understand than the latest thinking on nutrition. With **EAT THIS, NOT THAT!**, you're armed with the info you need to make smart choices. But how can you crank it up a notch? How can you make good nutrition as certain as death, taxes, and *Pirates of the Caribbean* spinoffs? Here's the simple answer: Just eat these eight foods—along with a little protein such as salmon, turkey, or lean beef—every day. And relax.

SPINACH

It may be green and leafy, but spinach is no nutritional wallflower. This noted muscle builder is a rich source of plant-based omega-3s and folate, which help reduce the risk of heart disease, stroke, and osteoporosis. Bonus: Folate also increases blood flow to the nether regions, helping to protect you against age-related sexual issues. And spinach is packed with lutein, a compound that fights macular degeneration. Aim for 1 cup fresh spinach or ½ cup cooked per day.
SUBSTITUTES: Kale, bok choy, romaine lettuce
FIT IT IN: Make your salads with spinach; add spinach to scrambled eggs; drape it over pizza; mix it with marinara sauce and then microwave for an instant dip.
PINCH HITTER: *Sesame Stir-Braised Kale* ❯ Heat 4 cloves minced garlic, 1 Tbsp. minced fresh ginger, and 1 tsp. sesame oil in a skillet. Add 2 Tbsp. water and 1 bunch kale (stemmed and chopped). Cover and cook for 3 minutes. Drain. Add 1 tsp. soy sauce and 1 Tbsp. sesame seeds.

YOGURT

Various cultures claim yogurt as their own creation, but the 2,000-year-old food's health benefits are not disputed: Fermentation spawns hundreds of millions of probiotic organisms that serve as reinforcements to the battalions of beneficial bacteria in your body. That helps boost your immune system and provides protection against cancer. Not all yogurts are probiotic, though, so make sure the label says "live and active cultures." Aim for 1 cup of the calcium- and protein-rich goop a day.

SUBSTITUTES: Kefir, soy yogurt

FIT IT IN: Yogurt topped with blueberries, walnuts, flaxseed, and honey is the ultimate breakfast—or dessert. Plain low-fat yogurt is also a perfect base for creamy salad dressings and dips.

HOME RUN: *Power Smoothie* > Blend 1 cup low-fat yogurt, 1 cup fresh or frozen blueberries, 1 cup carrot juice, and 1 cup fresh baby spinach for a nutrient-rich blast.

TOMATOES

There are two things you need to know about tomatoes: Red are the best, because they're packed with more of the antioxidant lycopene, and processed tomatoes are just as potent as fresh ones, because it's easier for the body to absorb the lycopene. Studies show that a diet rich in lycopene can decrease your risk of bladder, lung, prostate, skin, and stomach cancers, as well as reduce the risk of coronary artery disease. Aim for 22 mg of lycopene a day, which is about eight red cherry tomatoes or a glass of tomato juice.

SUBSTITUTES: Red watermelon, pink grapefruit, Japanese persimmon, papaya, guava

FIT IT IN: Pile on the ketchup and Ragú®; guzzle low-sodium V8® and gazpacho; double the amount of tomato paste called for in a recipe.

PINCH HITTER: *Red and Pink Fruit Bowl* > Chop 1 small watermelon, 2 grapefruits, and 1 papaya. Garnish with mint.

CARROTS

Most red, yellow, or orange vegetables and fruits are spiked with carotenoids—fat-soluble compounds that are associated with a reduction in a wide range of cancers, as well as reduced risk and severity of inflammatory conditions such as asthma and rheumatoid arthritis—but none are as easy to prepare, or have as low a caloric density, as carrots. Aim for $\frac{1}{2}$ cup a day.

SUBSTITUTES: Sweet potato, pumpkin, butternut squash, yellow bell pepper, mango

FIT IT IN: Raw baby carrots, sliced raw yellow pepper, butternut squash soup, baked sweet potato, pumpkin pie, mango sorbet, carrot cake

PINCH HITTER: *Baked Sweet Potato Fries* > Scrub and dry 2 sweet potatoes. Cut each into 8 slices, and then toss with olive oil and paprika. Spread on a baking sheet and bake for 15 minutes at 350°F. Turn and bake for 10 minutes more.

BLUEBERRIES

Host to more antioxidants than any other North American fruit, blueberries help prevent cancer, diabetes, and age-related memory changes (hence the nickname "brain berry"). Studies show that blueberries, which are rich in fiber and vitamins A and C, also boost cardiovascular health. Aim for 1 cup fresh blueberries a day, or $1/2$ cup frozen or dried.

SUBSTITUTES: Açai berries, purple grapes, prunes, raisins, strawberries

FIT IT IN: Blueberries maintain most of their power in dried, frozen, or jam form.

PINCH HITTER: Açai, an Amazonian berry, has even more antioxidants than the blueberry. Try açai juice from Sambazon® or add 2 Tbsp. of açai pulp to cereal, yogurt, or a smoothie.

BLACK BEANS

All beans are good for your heart, but none can boost your brain power like black beans. That's because they're full of anthocyanins, antioxidant compounds that have been shown to improve brain function. A daily $1/2$-cup serving provides 8 grams of protein and 7.5 grams of fiber. It's also low in calories and free of saturated fat.

SUBSTITUTES: Peas, lentils, and pinto, kidney, fava, and lima beans

FIT IT IN: Wrap black beans in a breakfast burrito; use both black beans and kidney beans in your chili; puree 1 cup black beans with $1/4$ cup olive oil and roasted garlic for a healthy dip; add favas, limas, or peas to pasta dishes.

HOME RUN: *Black Bean and Tomato Salsa* > Dice 4 tomatoes, 1 onion, 3 cloves garlic, 2 jalapeños, 1 yellow bell pepper, and 1 mango. Mix in a can of black beans and garnish with $1/2$ cup chopped cilantro and the juice of 2 limes.

WALNUTS

Richer in heart-healthy omega-3s than salmon, loaded with more anti-inflammatory polyphenols than red wine, and packing half as much muscle-building protein as chicken, the walnut sounds like a Frankenfood, but it grows on trees. Other nuts combine only one or two of these features, not all three. A serving of walnuts—about 1 ounce, or 7 nuts—is good anytime, but especially as a postworkout recovery snack.

SUBSTITUTES: Almonds, peanuts, pistachios, macadamia nuts, hazelnuts

FIT IT IN: Sprinkle on top of salads; chop and add to pancake batter; spoon peanut butter into curries; grind and mix with olive oil to make a marinade for grilled fish or chicken.

HOME RUN: Mix 1 cup walnuts with $\frac{1}{2}$ cup dried blueberries and $\frac{1}{4}$ cup dark chocolate chunks.

OATS

The *éminence grise* of health food, oats garnered the FDA's first seal of approval. They are packed with soluble fiber, which lowers the risk of heart disease. Yes, oats are loaded with carbs, but the release of those sugars is slowed by the fiber, and because oats also have 10 grams of protein per $\frac{1}{2}$-cup serving, they deliver steady, muscle-friendly energy.

SUBSTITUTES: Quinoa, flaxseed, wild rice

FIT IT IN: Eat granolas and cereals that have a fiber content of at least 5 grams per serving. Sprinkle 2 Tbsp. ground flaxseed on cereals, salads, and yogurt.

PINCH HITTER: *Quinoa Salad* ❯ Quinoa has twice the protein of most cereals, and fewer carbs. Boil 1 cup quinoa in 2 cups of water. Let cool. In a large bowl, toss it with 2 diced apples, 1 cup fresh blueberries, $\frac{1}{2}$ cup chopped walnuts, and 1 cup plain fat-free yogurt.

1,020 calories

Pepperidge Farm Roasted Chicken Pot Pie is the worst meal in your supermarket.

The 20 Worst Foods in America

The U.S. food industry has declared war on your waistline. Here's how to disarm its weapons of mass inflation

WORST FAST-FOOD CHICKEN MEAL

20 Chicken Selects® Premium Breast Strips from McDonald's (5 pieces) with creamy ranch sauce

830 calories
55 g fat (4.5 g trans fat)
48 g carbs

The only thing "premium" about these strips is the caloric price you pay. Add a large fries and regular soda and this seemingly innocuous chicken meal tops out at 1,710 calories.

Change Your Chicken 20 McNuggets® have the same impact. Instead, choose Mickey D's six-piece offering with BBQ sauce and save yourself 530 calories.

WORST DRINK

19 Jamba Juice Chocolate Moo'd® Power Smoothie (30 fl oz)

900 calories / 10 g fat
183 g carbs (166 g sugar)

Jamba Juice calls it a smoothie; we call it a milkshake. In fact, this beverage contains as much sugar as 2 pints of Ben and Jerry's Butter Pecan ice cream.

Turn Down the Power More than half of this chain's "power smoothies" contain in excess of 100 grams of sugar. Stick to Jamba's lower-calorie "All Fruit" smoothies, which are the only smoothies that contain no added sugar. And always opt for the 16-ounce "small."

WORST SUPERMARKET MEAL

18 Pepperidge Farm Roasted Chicken Pot Pie (whole pie)

1,020 calories / 64 g fat
86 g carbs

The label may say this pie serves two, but who ever divided a small pot pie in half? Once you crack the crust, there will be no stopping.

Pick a Better Pie Swanson's pot pie has just 400 calories.

WORST "HEALTHY" BURGER

17 Ruby Tuesday Bella Turkey Burger

1,145 calories / 71 g fat
56 g carbs

We chose this burger for more than its calorie payload: Its name implies that it's healthy.

The Truly Healthy Choice Skip burgers entirely (few at Ruby Tuesday come in under 1,000 calories). Instead, order a 7-ounce sirloin with a side of steamed vegetables.

GUT BOMBS TO GO

In an age of supersize combo meals, 17-syllable coffee drinks, and 6-inch-long ingredient lists, it's hard to know what, exactly, you're eating—especially when you're in a hurry. Here are six items you should do without.

The Worst... COFFEE

Starbucks Venti Strawberries and Crème Frappucino® Blended Crème

750 calories / 120 g sugars

Has more sugar than three cans of soda.
Say The Magic Word Order any blended drink "light" to cut the sugar in half.

DOUGHNUT

Krispy Kreme Caramel Kreme Crunch

380 calories
21 g fat (6 g trans fat)
46 g carbohydrates

At about four or five bites per doughnut, it may provide more calories per swallow than any other food.
Damage Control Krispy Kreme's Whole Wheat doughnut is the only one on the menu that contains less than 200 calories.

BREAKFAST SANDWICH

Dunkin' Donuts Sausage, Egg, and Cheese Croissant

630 calories
45 g fat

Contains nearly an entire day's worth of saturated fat. (Blame the croissant.)
A Perfect Portion The Ham, Egg, and Cheese English Muffin Sandwich packs a heavy dose of protein for a mere 310 calories.

MINIMART SNACK

Hostess Fruit Pie, Cherry

480 calories / 33 g sugars
20 g fat

There are trace amounts of real cherries, but they're hidden behind a wall of high-fructose corn syrup and refined flour.

AIRPORT SNACK

Cinnabon Classic Cinnamon Roll

813 calories
32 g fat (5 g trans fat)
117 g carbs

This roll may give you a sugar lift, but a crash will soon follow.
Walk Away You're better off hoofing it over to Burger King for a regular Whopper®, which contains 150 fewer calories but 13 more grams of protein. Just pass on the combo meal.

DRIVE-THRU COMBO MEAL

Burger King Triple Whopper® with Cheese, Fries, and Coke®, King-Size

2,200 calories
115 g fat (11 g trans fat)
225 g carbs / (117 g sugars)
2,590 mg sodium

Contains more carbs than 10 bread slices.
Create Your Own Combo The Angus Steak Burger, garden side salad, and your choice of diet drink can fill you up for a justifiable 660 calories.

813 calories
What sugar crashes are made of.

8

16 Chipotle Mexican Grilled Chicken Burrito

1,107 calories / 44 g fat
113 g carbs
2,656 mg sodium

Despite a reputation for using healthy, fresh ingredients, Chipotle's menu is limited to king-size burritos, overstuffed tacos, and gigantic salads—all of which lead to a humongous waistline. **Make Over the Menu** There are two ways to make a Chipotle burrito healthy enough to eat: (1) 86 the rice and tortilla and request your meat, vegetables, and beans served in a bowl, or (2) bring a friend and saw the burrito in half.

15 Macaroni Grill Double Macaroni 'n' Cheese

1,210 calories / 62 g fat
3,450 mg sodium

It's like feeding your kid 1½ boxes of Kraft mac 'n' cheese. **Your Best Option** The 390-calorie Grilled Chicken and Broccoli.

14 Quizno's Chicken Carbonara (large)

1,510 calories / 82 g fat
106 g carbs / 3,750 mg sodium

A large homemade sandwich would more likely provide about 500 calories. **Cut the Calories** Isn't it obvious? Order a small—or save half for later.

13 On the Border Grande Taco Salad with Taco Beef

1,450 calories / 102 g fat
78 g carbs / 2,410 mg sodium

This isn't an anomaly: Five different On the Border salads on the menu contain more than 1,100 calories each. **The Salad for You** The Sizzling Chicken Fajita Salad supplies an acceptable 760 calories.But remember to choose a noncaloric beverage, such as water or unsweetened iced tea.

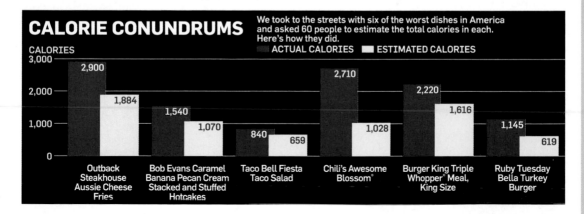

CALORIE CONUNDRUMS

We took to the streets with six of the worst dishes in America and asked 60 people to estimate the total calories in each. Here's how they did.

■ ACTUAL CALORIES ■ ESTIMATED CALORIES

	ACTUAL	ESTIMATED
Outback Steakhouse Aussie Cheese Fries	2,900	1,884
Bob Evans Caramel Banana Pecan Cream Stacked and Stuffed Hotcakes	1,540	1,070
Taco Bell Fiesta Taco Salad	840	659
Chili's Awesome Blossom	2,710	1,028
Burger King Triple Whopper Meal, King Size	2,220	1,616
Ruby Tuesday Bella Turkey Burger	1,145	619

CALORIES: 3,000 — 2,000 — 1,000 — 0

WORST BURGER

12 Carl's Jr. Double Six Dollar Burger®

1,520 calories / 111 g fat

Carl's brags about this, but also provides convenient nutrition info on its Web site—so ignorance is no excuse for eating it. **A Simple Solution** The Low Carb Six Dollar Burger® has just 490 calories.

WORST STEAK

11 Lonestar 20 oz T-bone

1,540 calories / 124 g fat

Add a baked potato and Lonestar's Signature Lettuce Wedge, and this is a 2,700-calorie blowout. **Make the Cut** Stick to fillets and sirloins in steakhouses— they're the two leanest cuts of beef.

WORST BREAKFAST

10 Bob Evans Caramel Banana Pecan Cream Stacked and Stuffed Hotcakes

1,540 calories
77 g fat (9 g trans fat)
198 g carbs (109 g sugar)

Five Egg McMuffins® yield the same caloric cost as these sugar-stuffed flapjacks. **Order This Instead** The Western Omelet has 654 calories and 44 grams of protein.

WORST DESSERT

9 Chili's Chocolate Chip Paradise Pie with Vanilla Ice Cream

1,600 calories / 78 g fat
215 g carbs

Would you eat a Big Mac for dessert? How about three? That's the calorie equivalent of this decadent dish. Clearly, Chili's customers get their money's worth. **Don't Overdo It** If you want dessert at Chili's, order one single-serving Sweet Shot; you'll cap your after-dinner intake at 310 calories.

WORST CHINESE ENTRÉE

8 P.F. Chang's Pork Lo Mein

1,820 calories / 127 g fat
95 g carbs

The fat content in this dish alone provides more than 1,100 calories. And you'd have to eat almost five servings of pasta to match the number of carbohydrates it contains. Now, do you really need five servings of pasta? **Pick Another Noodle** P.F. Chang's Singapore Street Noodles will satisfy your craving with only 570 calories. Or try the Moo Goo Gai Pan or the Ginger Chicken & Broccoli, which have 660 calories each.

RESTAURANT REPORT CARD

No one expects restaurants to serve only healthy fare. But they should provide options. So to separate the commendable from the deplorable, we calculated the total number of calories per entrée in 21 fast-food and sit-down chains. This gave us a snapshot of how each restaurant compared in average serving size—a key indicator of unhealthy portion distortion. Then we rewarded establishments with fruit and vegetable side-dish choices, as well as offering whole wheat bread. Finally, we penalized places for excessive amounts of trans fats and menus laden with gut-busting desserts. Did your favorite restaurant make the grade?

FAST-FOOD RESTAURANTS

Chick-Fil-A
Not a single sandwich breaks the 500-calorie barrier, a feat unmatched in the fast-food world. **A+**

Subway
An impressive selection of 6-inch sandwiches with less than 400 calories each earns Jared's joint a second-place finish. **A**

Boston Market
Its expansive menu of healthy sides and nutritionally reasonable three-piece chicken meals gives diners plenty of choices. **A-**

Taco Bell
It's okay to "make a run for the border," as long as you limit yourself to just two tacos or a single burrito. **B+**

Wendy's
Although calorically comparable to McDonald's, Wendy's edges out the Arches with less trans fat and a range of healthy sides. **B**

McDonald's
Burgers are reasonable, but others, like pancake platters, send McDonald's numbers soaring. **B-**

KFC
It's hard to have "fried" in your name and still make a decent grade. To halve calories, order your chicken without skin. **C+**

Arby's
The array of sandwiches suffers from an abundance of creamy dressings, spreads, and melted cheese sauce. **C**

Burger King
Thousand-calorie-plus burgers like the Quad Stacker give this chain a below-average score. **C-**

Domino's
Two slices of any Feast pizza contain from 460 (thin-crust vegetable) to 880 calories (MeatZZa, deep dish). **C-**

Panera
Healthy sides, whole grains, and free Wi-Fi can't offset oversized, calorie-loaded salads and sandwiches. **D**

Pizza Hut
Massive pasta portions are nearly 1,000 calories, while personal pan pizzas average 660 calories. **D-**

SIT-DOWN RESTAURANTS

Bob Evans
A massive menu of reasonable egg dishes and extensive sides ranging from broccoli to applesauce boosts Bob to the top spot. **A-**

Fazoli's
Pasta portions are thankfully restrained and can be topped with chicken, broccoli, and tomatoes, or garlic shrimp. **B+**

Denny's
Abysmal burgers and the carb-loaded Grand Slams® are offset by a range of lighter alternatives on the Fit Fare menu. **B**

Ruby Tuesday
Most of the burgers hover around the 1,000-calorie mark, but seafood and chicken options offer a shot at redemption. **B-**

Uno Chicago Grill
Any meal involving deep-dish pizza will likely break the 1,000-calorie barrier. (Go with a flatbread pizza.) **C**

Chili's
Monster burgers and 2,000-calorie starters hurt. Order from the Guiltless Grill menu to keep your calorie intake under 650. **C-**

P.F. Chang's
Most entrées begin in a wok with a puddle of oil and a scoop of sugar- and salt-laden sauce. Hunt for steamed options instead. **D**

On the Border
An average "Favorito" entrée contains 1,000-plus calories. Stick to two tacos and a side of grilled vegetables. **F**

Macaroni Grill
Even lunch portions and salads have more than 1,000 calories. Either split a pasta or order the 330-calorie Pollo Magro. **F**

Minimum Disclosure Sure, Macaroni Grill earns its F with a menu full of 1,500-calorie pastas, but at least it provides nutritional information to its customers. We contacted the following restaurants and asked them to give up their full nutritional numbers, but all 15 refused.
Applebee's, Bonefish Grill, California Pizza Kitchen, Chipotle, Cracker Barrel, Fuddruckers, Hooters, IHOP, Maggiano's Little Italy, Olive Garden, Outback, Perkins, Ruth's Chris Steakhouse, T.G.I. Friday's
NOTE: We were able to obtain nutritional data for some dishes from the Center for Science in the Public Interest and CalorieKing.com.
LAUREN MURROW

7 Chili's Honey Chipotle Crispers with Chipotle Sauce

2,040 calories / 99 g fat 240 g carbs

"Crispers" refers to an extra-thick layer of bread crumbs that soaks up oil and adds unnecessary calories and carbs to these glorified chicken strips.

Switch Your Selection Order the Chicken Fajita Pita: At 450 calories and 43 grams of protein, it's one of the healthiest entrées you'll find in a chain restaurant.

6 On the Border Dos XX® Fish Tacos with Rice and Beans

2,100 calories / 130 g fat 169 g carbs / 4,750 mg sodium

Perhaps the most misleadingly named dish in America: A dozen crunchy tacos from Taco Bell will saddle you with fewer calories.

Lighten the Load Ask for grilled fish, choose the corn tortillas instead of flour (they're lower in calories and higher in fiber), and swap out the carbohydrate-loaded rice for grilled vegetables.

5 Uno Chicago Grill Chicago Classic Deep Dish Pizza

2,310 calories / 162 g fat 123 g carbs / 4,470 mg sodium

Downing this "personal" pizza is equivalent to eating 18 slices of Domino's Crunchy Thin Crust cheese pizza.

Swap Your Slices Switch to the Sausage Flatbread Pie and avert deep-dish disaster by nearly 1,500 calories.

4 Macaroni Grill Spaghetti and Meatballs with Meat Sauce

2,430 calories / 128 g fat 207 g carbs / 5,290 mg sodium

This meal satisfies your calorie requirements for an entire day.

Downsize the Devastation Ask for a lunch portion of this dinner dish (or any pasta on the menu, for that matter), and request regular tomato sauce instead of meat sauce. You'll cut the calories in half.

3 On the Border Stacked Border Nachos

2,740 calories / 166 g fat 191 g carbs / 5,280 mg sodium

2 Chili's Awesome Blossom®

2,710 calories / 203 g fat 194 g carbs / 6,360 mg sodium

1 Outback Steakhouse Aussie Cheese Fries® with Ranch Dressing

2,900 calories / 182 g fat 240 g carbs

Even if you split these "starters" with three friends, you'll have downed a dinner's worth of calories before your entrée arrives.

Super Substitutions Front-load your meal with a protein-based dish that's not deep-fried. A high-protein starter helps diminish hunger without putting you into calorie overload. And remember: Appetizers are meant to be shared.

At On the Border:
Chicken Soft Tacos (250 calories each). This entrée is as close as you'll come to a healthy starter.

At Chili's:
Garlic & Lime Grilled Shrimp. Look for this item in the "sides."

At Outback:
Seared Ahi or Shrimp on the Barbie.

2,900 calories
Outback's Aussie
Cheese Fries®:
The Worst Food
in America.

Chapter 2

AT YOUR FAVORITE RESTAURANTS

Applebee's

Did You Know?

● Applebee's has restaurants in 18 countries, including such unlikely homes for the "neighborhood bar and grill" as Qatar and Bahrain.

● Applebee's completed a three-year transition to fry and grill all foods in a blend of soybean oils in the spring of 2007, ridding its menu of trans fats.

GUILTY PLEASURE

Onion Soup Au Gratin

150 calories
8 g fat

French onion soup is usually coated in oozing cheese and loaded in fat, but this updated version is packed with caramelized onions and subs a layer of reduced-fat cheese.

Eat This

Grilled Cajun Lime Tilapia

with Black Bean & Corn Salsa

310 calories
6 g fat
(0 g saturated)
1,250 mg sodium*

Just a few ounces of fish a week can cut heart attack risk by 38 percent, according to a Greek study.

Get all the same lively Southwestern flavors as Fiesta Lime Chicken for a quarter of the calories.

Other Picks

Crispy Buttermilk Shrimp
with potatoes and toast

843 calories
34 g fat (9 g saturated)
1,563 mg sodium

Teriyaki Steak & Shrimp Skewers

370 calories
7 g fat (2 g saturated)
1,475 mg sodium

1,285 calories
47 g fat
(14 g saturated)
1,443 mg sodium

Not That!

Fiesta Lime Chicken®

with Sauce, Cheese, Tortilla Strips, Salsa, Rice

*Numbers are approximate; Applebee's does not provide nutrition information.

Even though the chicken is grilled rather than fried, a coating of ranch and cheddar sauce and a handful of tortilla strips boosts the fat content.

HIDDEN DANGER

Low-Fat Chicken Quesadillas

This may seem like a healthy alternative to burgers and fried food, but the collective impact of calories and carbs will do its best to stretch you horizontally.

742 calories
14 g fat
86 g carbohydrates

LITTLE TRICK

Sub healthy sides like steamed broccoli or mixed vegetables for the garlic toast that accompanies most sandwiches and salads. The buttery toast tacks on 7 grams of fat with zero nutritional value.

Other Passes

1,295 calories
82 g fat (26 g saturated)
2,199 mg sodium

Grilled Steak Caesar Salad
with toast

1,605 calories
121 g fat (38 g saturated)
2,330 mg sodium

Southwest Philly Roll-Up
with salsa

Arby's

Did You Know?

● Arby's was the first major fast food restaurant in the U.S. to eliminate trans fats from their menu.

● Arby's roast beef is slow-cooked in the store for 4 hours. Like most supermarket roast beefs, though, Arby's injects theirs with water, salt, and preservatives.

LITTLE TRICK

Avoid any sandwich made on honey wheat bread: Two slices contain a staggering 361 calories and 68 grams of carbs. Cut those in half by sticking to a sesame seed bun.

Eat This

Super Roast Beef

440 calories
19 g fat
(7 g saturated)
1,061 mg sodium

Replacing some of the carbohydrates in your diet with red meat can lower blood pressure. This sandwich combines roast beef, tomatoes, and lettuce, and replaces mayo with a low-cal spicy pepper sauce.

Other Picks

Chicken Cordon Bleu Sandwich— Grilled

488 calories
18 g fat (4 g saturated)
1,560 mg sodium

Martha's Vineyard Salad™
with Light Buttermilk Ranch Dressing

389 calories
14 g fat (5 g saturated)
923 mg sodium

810 calories
42 g fat
(13 g saturated)
1,780 mg sodium

Not That!

Roast Beef and Swiss Market Fresh® Sandwich

They look and sound the same, right? But the unwholesome trinity of mayo, Italian sub sauce, and processed Swiss cheese make the sandwich the clear loser in the battle of the beef.

Other Passes

769 calories
39 g fat (10 g saturated)
1,240 mg sodium

Chicken Salad with Pecans Sandwich

773 calories
52 g fat (10 g saturated)
1,823 mg sodium

Santa Fe Salad™
with Santa Fe Ranch Dressing

WEAPON OF MASS DESTRUCTION

Large Mozzarella Sticks

The Impact:
849 calories
56 g fat (26 g saturated)
2,730 mg sodium
As much saturated fat as a Triple Whopper®.

MENU DECODER

● **CHICKEN NATURALS®:** The FDA has no definition of "all natural," so chains like Arby's can serve "100% all-natural chicken" despite using artificial flavoring.

● **CIABATTA:** A small, airy Italian loaf often used to make panini in upscale sandwich shops. Here, the fancy bread comes with a price: 305 calories and 60 grams of carbohydrates.

19

Did You Know?

● The company's motto is "the sun never rises twice on our bread." Left-over bakery items are donated to local charities on a daily basis.

● Breakfast items pack a punch: Omelets and croissant sandwiches all have more than 20 grams of fat. Stick to scrambled eggs.

LITTLE TRICK

Ask for your sandwich on lower-carb multigrain bread. It will save you 180 calories and 42 grams of carbohydrates over the next best pick, the whole wheat.

Eat This

Roasted Turkey Breast

on Nine Grain without cheese or mayo

430 calories
7 g fat
(2 g saturated)
1,350 mg sodium

Ordering this sandwich sans cheese and mayo slices 21 grams of fat from your lunch.

Other Picks

Spicy Chicken Gumbo

120 calories
2.5 g fat (0 g saturated)
1,460 mg sodium

Banana Nut Bread

230 calories
14 g fat (1.5 g saturated)
120 mg sodium

Tall Cappuccino

130 calories
5 g fat (3 g saturated)
135 mg sodium

Not That!

California Avocado
on Tomato Onion Focaccia without cheese

690 calories
40 g fat
(7 g saturated)
1,010 mg sodium

The bread this sandwich is served on delivers 920 mg of sodium and 6 grams of fat on its own. Sub thinner sliced bread for carb-heavy focaccia.

Other Passes

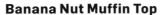

290 calories
18 g fat (6 g saturated)
1,340 mg sodium

Homestyle Chicken and Dumplings

420 calories
26 g fat (3 g saturated)
190 mg sodium

Banana Nut Muffin Top

450 calories
10 g fat (6 g saturated)
230 mg sodium

Tall Hot Chocolate

MENU DECODER

● **PASTA PUTTANESCA:** Penne pasta topped with a tomato sauce spiked with capers, olives, and fresh basil—the healthiest of ABC's pasta choices by far.

● **FOCCACIA:** A round loaf made from dough similar to a pizza crust, seasoned with olive oil and herbs and topped with cheese, onions, or tomatoes.

HIDDEN DANGER

Bran Raisin Muffin

"Bran" and "Raisin" don't translate into the nutritional equivalent of Raisin Bran. Nearly half of the calories in a typical large muffin come from fat—basically the same recipe as cake.

410 calories
18 g fat
(2.5 g saturated)
30 g sugars

21

Auntie Anne's

● At this popular mall snack stop, pretzel dough is mixed, rolled by hand, and baked fresh every 30 minutes on site. All told, Auntie Anne's bakers make 100 million pretzels per year (using enough dough in the process to wrap end-to-end around the earth three times).

LITTLE TRICK

Order your pretzel without salt and the sodium drops from 930 mg to about 500 mg. Order without butter, and you'll lose two grams of saturated fat and up to 60 calories.

Eat This

Jalapeño Pretzel

without Butter w/ Marinara Sauce

280 calories
1.5 g fat
(0 g saturated)
960 mg sodium

This pretzel/dip combo is the lowest-calorie option on the menu.

Other Picks

Original Pretzel without Butter
with Sweet Pretzel Dip

380 calories
4 g fat (2 g saturated)
900 mg sodium

Blue Raspberry Dutch Ice®
14 oz

165 calories
0 g fat
37 g sugars

22

450 calories
9.5 g fat
(4 g saturated)
1,610 mg sodium

Not That!

Whole Wheat Pretzel

without Butter w/ Cheese Sauce

WEAPON OF MASS DESTRUCTION

Strawberry Dutch Shake (20 oz)

The Impact:
910 calories, 41 g fat
(26 g saturated fat)
110 g sugars

Make it a Strawberry Dutch Ice and save 595 calories and 26 grams of fat

The Whole Wheat Pretzel supplies 7 grams of fiber, as much as a cup of bran cereal. Unfortunately, it also has a higher sodium content than any other pretzel on the menu, at 1,120 mg.

DIP DECODER

● **MARINARA SAUCE:** 30 calories, 0 g fat

● **SWEET DIP:** 40 calories, 0 g fat

● **SWEET MUSTARD:** 60 calories, 1.5 g fat

● **CARAMEL DIP:** 135 calories, 3 g fat

● **LIGHT CREAM CHEESE:** 70 calories, 6 g fat

● **CHEESE SAUCE:** 100 calories, 8 g fat

Other Passes

540 calories
6.5 g fat (4 g saturated)
600 mg sodium

Glazin' Raisin® Pretzel
without Butter with Light Cream Cheese

400 calories
10 g fat (9 g saturated)
52 g sugars

Mocha Dutch Ice®
14 oz

23

Au Bon Pain

Did You Know?

● Au Bon Pain is French for "on good bread." The salad and sandwich spot (found in airports across the country) makes all its breads by hand with organic flour and French sea salt. Artisan or not, two slices of French country white bread still has 260 calories and 54 grams of carbohydrates.

GUILTY PLEASURE

Portobello and Goat Cheese Sandwich

540 calories,
27 g fat (8 g saturated)

Mushrooms are packed with selenium. Harvard researchers found that men with the highest levels of selenium had a 48 percent lower incidence of advanced prostate cancer.

Eat This

Thai Peanut Chicken Wrap

630 calories
6 g fat
(2 g saturated)
1,070 mg sodium

Field greens, tomato, cucumber, and carrots deliver vitamins to help protect your heart and prevent cell damage.

Other Picks

Jamaican Black Bean Soup
(medium)

180 calories
1 g fat (0 g saturated)
460 mg sodium

Small Vanilla Yogurt
with Granola and Blueberries

310 calories
6 g fat (2 g saturated)
130 mg sodium

Not That!

Turkey and Swiss Sandwich

850 calories
41 g fat
(14 g saturated)
1,640 mg sodium

A combination of Swiss cheese and creamy dressing pushes the fat and sodium levels through the roof.

WEAPON OF MASS DESTRUCTION

Sausage, Egg, & Cheddar on an Asiago Bagel

770 calories
36 g fat (17 g saturated)
1,620 mg sodium

Start your morning with this gut bomb and be confined to eating rice cakes the rest of the day.

MENU DECODER

● **ASIAGO:**
An Italian cow's milk cheese that can be either soft and smooth, or hard and crumbly like Parmesan, depending on the age of the cheese. Most often found in the U.S. baked into breads, where it adds an extra dose of fat and sodium (and a token bit of protein) to whatever it touches.

Other Passes

290 calories
16 g fat (5 g saturated)
930 mg sodium

Chicken Vegetable Stew
(medium)

570 calories
36 g fat (13 g saturated)
270 mg sodium

Almond Croissant

Baja Fresh

Did You Know?

● Baja Fresh doesn't own a microwave, freezer, or a can opener in any of its 300+ locations. This Cali chain prides itself on preparing everything—from the half-dozen salsas to the grilled, marinated meats—fresh on site.

● Baja goes heavy on the salt. Few of the entrées on the menu have under 2,000 mg of sodium. Your strategy? Stick with the tacos and salads, preferably with shrimp or fish. And whenever possible, choose corn tortillas over flour—they're much lower in sodium.

Eat This

Two Grilled Mahi Mahi Tacos

460 calories
18 g fat
(3 g saturated)
600 mg sodium

The fish in fish tacos is traditionally battered and fried. The grilled version provides the heart-healthy benefits of fish without the oil-sponge coat.

By skipping the complimentary basket of chips, you save 210 calories and 9 grams of fat.

Other Picks

Baja Ensalada
with Charbroiled Chicken with salsa

325 calories
7 g fat (2 g saturated)
1,580 mg sodium

2 Original Baja Carnitas Tacos

440 calories
14 g fat (4 g saturated)
560 mg sodium

950 calories
44 g fat
(**21** g saturated)
2,310 mg sodium

Not That!
Steak Burrito Ultimo®

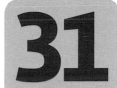

31

Grams of fat you cut from your salad when you dress it with Salsa Verde instead of olive oil vinaigrette

Order "bare style" and Baja will serve your burrito in a bowl, saving you about 300 calories.

MENU DECODER

● **SALSA VERDE:**
Mild "green sauce" made from roasted tomatillos, onions, cilantro, and lime

● **COTIJA CHEESE:**
Crumbly Mexican cheese with a flavor similar to feta used to top salads and beans.

● **CARNITAS:**
Traditionally, pork slow-cooked in lard. Luckily, at Baja, they stew their pork in a bath of chicken stock, onions, garlic, and herbs.

Other Passes

1,140 calories
55 g fat (**14** g saturated)
2,370 mg sodium

Charbroiled Chicken Tostada

1,190 calories
43 g fat (**14** g saturated)
3,450 mg sodium

Carnitas Fajitas
with Flour Tortillas

Baskin-Robbins

Did You Know?

● The "31" in Baskin-Robbins 31 Flavors stands for a different ice cream flavor for every day of the month. The chain has created more than 1,000 flavors since 1945.

LITTLE TRICK

Baskin-Robbins offers four flavors of low-fat ice cream and seven flavors of low-fat or nonfat frozen yogurt. Try to avoid ice creams with caramel or chocolate "ribbons" swirled in to cut back on sugar—they're made mostly of high-fructose corn syrup.

Eat This

2-Scoop Hot Fudge Sundae

Chocolate and Vanilla

530 calories
29 g fat
(19 g saturated)
52 g sugars

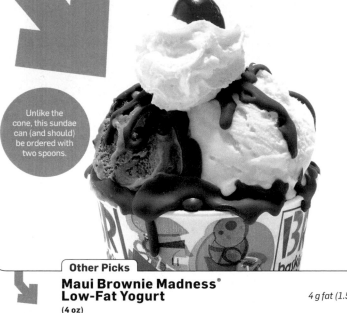

Unlike the cone, this sundae can (and should) be ordered with two spoons.

Other Picks

Maui Brownie Madness® Low-Fat Yogurt
(4 oz)

210 calories
4 g fat (1.5 g saturated)
34 g sugars

Cherries Jubilee Ice Cream
(4 oz)

240 calories
12 fat (7 g saturated)
26 g sugars

Caramel Turtle Ice Cream
(4 oz, no sugar added, low-fat)

160 calories
4 g fat (3 g saturated)
7 g sugars

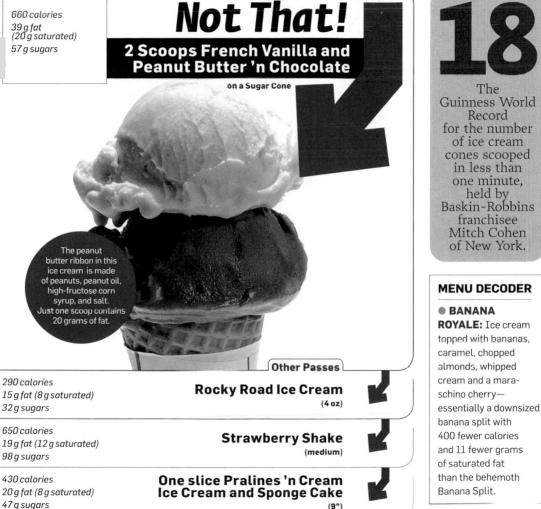

660 calories
39 g fat
(20 g saturated)
57 g sugars

Not That!

2 Scoops French Vanilla and Peanut Butter 'n Chocolate

on a Sugar Cone

The peanut butter ribbon in this ice cream is made of peanuts, peanut oil, high-fructose corn syrup, and salt. Just one scoop contains 20 grams of fat.

18

The Guinness World Record for the number of ice cream cones scooped in less than one minute, held by Baskin-Robbins franchisee Mitch Cohen of New York.

MENU DECODER

● **BANANA ROYALE:** Ice cream topped with bananas, caramel, chopped almonds, whipped cream and a maraschino cherry— essentially a downsized banana split with 400 fewer calories and 11 fewer grams of saturated fat than the behemoth Banana Split.

Other Passes

290 calories
15 g fat (8 g saturated)
32 g sugars

Rocky Road Ice Cream
(4 oz)

650 calories
19 g fat (12 g saturated)
98 g sugars

Strawberry Shake
(medium)

430 calories
20 g fat (8 g saturated)
47 g sugars

One slice Pralines 'n Cream Ice Cream and Sponge Cake
(9")

Ben & Jerry's

Did You Know?

● All of B&J's dairy comes from Vermont dairy farmers who have pledged not to treat their cows with Recombinant Bovine Growth Hormone (rBGH).

● Ben & Jerry's ensures their pints have the right amount of mix-ins by melting them down in a strainer and washing off the ice cream, then weighing the chunks.

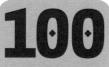

100

Number of gallons sacrificed daily for quality control

Eat This

Strawberry Kiwi Swirl Sorbet

and Berry Berry Extraordinary® Sorbet in a Sugar Cone (½ cup each)

280 calories
1 g fat
(0 g saturated)
52 g sugars

Sorbet may be as sugar-packed as ice cream, but it's dairy- and fat-free.

Other Picks

Chocolate Fudge Brownie™ Frozen Yogurt
(½ cup)

190 calories
2.5 g fat (1.5 g saturated)
23 g sugars

Strawberry Original Ice Cream
(½ cup)

230 calories
13 g fat (9 g saturated)
25 g sugars

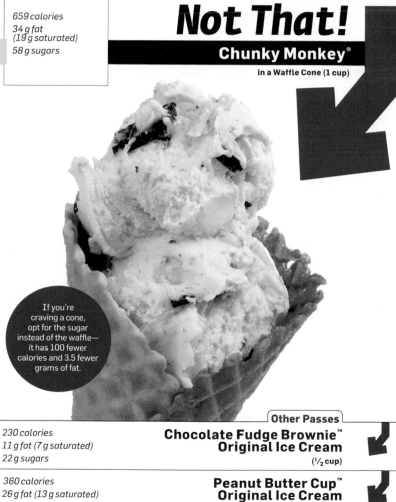

659 calories
34 g fat
(19 g saturated)
58 g sugars

Not That!

Chunky Monkey®

in a Waffle Cone (1 cup)

If you're craving a cone, opt for the sugar instead of the waffle—it has 100 fewer calories and 3.5 fewer grams of fat.

Other Passes

230 calories
11 g fat (7 g saturated)
22 g sugars

Chocolate Fudge Brownie™ Original Ice Cream
(½ cup)

360 calories
26 g fat (13 g saturated)
23 g sugars

Peanut Butter Cup™ Original Ice Cream
(½ cup)

LITTLE TRICK

Order smooth flavors rather than those mixed with baked or candy pieces. Flavors with chunks like peanut butter cups, Heath bars, or cookie dough contain heavy doses of hydrogenated fat. The healthiest regular scoops are strawberry, coffee, and vanilla, respectively.

MENU DECODER

● **CHOCOLATE LIQUOR:** The flavoring in some of Ben & Jerry's ice creams like Brownie Batter and Chubby Hubby®. It's created when cocoa nibs are ground to a fine liquid above the melting point of cocoa butter. Despite the name's boozy implications, chocolate liquor is nonalcoholic.

BLIMPIE

Did You Know?

● BLIMPIE's cookies are made with partially hydrogenated oils. Each contains anywhere from 1 to 5 grams of harmful trans fats.

● The "seasoning" for the Cream of Potato soup includes partially hydrogenated coconut oil, corn syrup, and bacon fat.

LITTLE TRICK

Skip the roll and order your sandwich on Mediterranean Flatbread to avoid the high-fructose corn syrup and partially hydrogenated oils that are contained in most BLIMPIE breads.

Eat This

Grilled Chicken Sub
(6" regular) and Seafood Salad

456 calories
10 g fat
(2 g saturated)
1,260 mg sodium

The wrap isn't always the healthier option; a six-inch white sub roll has 5 fewer grams of fat and 12 fewer grams of carbs than the Chicken Caesar's spinach herb tortilla, which contains partially hydrogenated oils.

Other Picks

Tomato Basil with Raviolini Soup and Tossed Salad
with fat-free Italian dressing

165 calories
3 g fat (1 g saturated)
1,379 mg sodium

Bluffin™ with Egg and Cheese

245 calories
10 g fat (5 g saturated)
771 mg sodium

Lay's KC Masterpiece® BBQ Flavored Potato Chips
(1 bag)

135 calories
3 g fat (0 g saturated)
236 g sodium

937 calories
51 g fat
(14 g saturated)
2,376 mg sodium

Not That!

Chicken Caesar Wrap

and Macaroni Salad

A seemingly low-fat choice is slathered in Caesar dressing, which contributes 21 grams of fat and 4 grams of saturated fat. The same goes for macaroni drenched in a creamy sauce made of mayo and corn syrup.

WEAPON OF MASS DESTRUCTION

12-inch Italian Style Meatball Sub, "stacked"

The Impact:
1,458 calories
78 g fat (37 g saturated; 2 g trans fat)
3,975 mg sodium

"Stacked" means it comes loaded with double the meat and cheese of the regular size. A six-inch version of this meaty monstrosity would still deliver 95 percent of your daily allotment of saturated fat.

Other Passes

423 calories
15 g fat (4 g saturated)
1,300 mg sodium

Chicken Soup with White and Wild Rice
with a Honey Oat roll (4")

495 calories
35 g fat (13 g saturated; 3 g trans fat)
1,118 mg sodium

Croissant with Egg, Sausage & Cheese

327 calories
17 g fat (5 g saturated; 5 g trans fat)
24 g sugars

Sugar Cookie

MENU DECODER

● **BLUFFIN™:** Blimpie's English muffin, served with cheese, ham, sausage, or bacon

● **BLIMPIE SPECIAL SUB DRESSING:** Vinegar, soybean oil, water, and artificial coloring

33

Bob Evans

34

Did You Know?

● Bob Evans first made his name selling pork sausage, and many of the items on the menu still carry the stuff. Before you rush for a taste, though, consider this: Three small links have more fat than a Big Mac.

MENU DECODER

● **EGG BEATERS®:**
A substitute for whole eggs composed of egg whites that have been fortified with other nutrients, including beta carotene, which gives them their yellow egg color. Egg Beaters® are higher in protein and free of fat and cholesterol.

Eat This

3 Scrambled Egg Beaters® Eggs

2 Slices Bacon, and Fresh Fruit

314 calories
19.5 g fat
(5 g saturated)
700 mg sodium

Cut 5 grams of fat and tack on 8 grams of protein by choosing Egg Beaters® over regular eggs.

Other Picks

Salmon
with Garlic Butter, Rice Pilaf, and Glazed Carrots

529 calories
23 g fat (6 g saturated)
1,071 mg sodium

Steak Tips
with Garden Vegetables

399 calories
23 g fat (6.5 g saturated)
1,039 mg sodium

Heritage Chef Salad
with Hot Bacon Dressing

365 calories
17.5 g fat (8 g saturated)
980 mg sodium

856 calories
19 g fat
(7 g saturated)
1,646 mg sodium

Not That!

2 Multigrain Hotcakes

with Syrup

No "multigrain" could possibly make up for 160 grams of carbohydrates found in this breakfast. One of the worst ways to start your day.

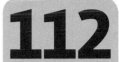

112

Number of minutes you would have to swim in rough surf to burn the 952 calories (and 80 grams of fat!) in one Bob Evans Bacon and Cheese Omelet.

HIDDEN DANGER

Cranberry Pecan Chicken Salad

Cranberries. Chicken. Pecans. Sounds healthy, right? Not when they're bound together by a bucket of mayonnaise and salt.

Other Passes

839 calories
38 g fat (12.5 g saturated)
1,608 mg sodium

Crispy Fish Sandwich

778 calories
45 g fat (18 g saturated)
2,588 mg sodium

Garden Vegetable Alfredo

700 calories
52.5 g fat (11 g saturated)
1,428 mg sodium

Country Spinach Salad
with Honey Mustard Dressing

800 calories
47 g fat
(15 g saturated)
1,949 mg sodium

Boston Market

Did You Know?

● Boston Market offers takeout meals for the holidays. According to the National Restaurant Association, 53 percent of Americans rely on takeout for part or all of their Thanksgiving dinners.

WEAPON OF MASS DESTRUCTION

Boston Meatloaf Carver

The Impact:
940 calories
45 g fat (18 g saturated)
2,080 mg sodium

More saturated fat than 30 Chicken McNuggets® and enough salt to preserve a small city.

Eat This

Roasted Sirloin, Garlic Dill New Potatoes, and Spinach

with Garlic Sauce

560 calories
27 g fat
(13 g saturated)
760 mg sodium

Lean beef is one of the richest sources of zinc, a key mineral in your immune system's fight against everything from viruses to cancer.

At just 290 calories a serving, the sirloin is one of the healthiest entrées at Boston Market

Other Picks

Roast Turkey, Broccoli
with Garlic Butter, and Butternut Squash

400 calories
13.5 g fat (6 g saturated)
900 mg sodium

Boston Turkey Carver

770 calories
27 g fat (8 g saturated)
1,810 mg sodium

Green Bean Casserole

60 calories
2 g fat (1 g saturated)
620 mg sodium

1,410 calories
90 g fat
(22 g saturated)
3020 mg sodium

Not That!

3 Pieces Dark Rotisserie Chicken

Sweet Potato Casserole, and Market Chopped Side Salad

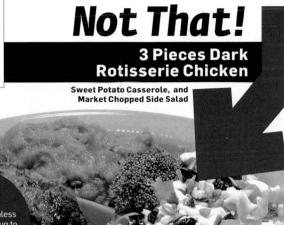

Ordering your chicken skinless instead can save up to 200 calories and 17 grams of fat.

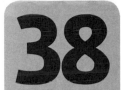

38

Grams of fat in the Caesar dressing. Dress your salad with Lite Ranch instead: It'll save you 34 grams of fat.

MENU DECODER

● **MARKET CHOPPED SALAD DRESSING:** A fatty blend of soybean oil, white wine vinegar, Dijon mustard, and honey. A single serving has 39 grams of fat.

GUILTY PLEASURE

Garden Fresh Cole Slaw

170 calories
9 g fat (2 g saturated)

Sure, there's a bit of mayo here, but cabbage is the top supplier of sulforaphane, a chemical that boosts your body's cancer-fighting enzymes.

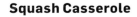
Other Passes

780 calores
47 g fat (17 g saturated)
930 mg sodium

Pastry Top Chicken Pot Pie

1,020 calories
51 g fat (15 g saturated)
2,450 mg sodium

Boston Sirloin Dip Carver Au Jus

320 calories
24 g fat (11 g saturated)
1,380 mg sodium

Squash Casserole

Burger King

Did You Know?

● In May of 2007, the Center for Science in the Public Interest sued Burger King for moving too slowly to remove trans fats from its menus. Less than two months later, Burger King responded with a promise to phase out all trans fats from its restaurants by the end of 2008.

MENU DECODER

● **GRILL FLAVOR:** An ingredient in some Burger King items, like the TENDERGRILL® Chicken Sandwich and the breakfast sausage. The "flavor" is actually partially hydrogenated soybean oil.

Eat This

WHOPPER JR®. without Mayo
and Garden Salad

365 calories
12 g fat
(4.5 g saturated)
1,230 mg sodium

You could eat 3 of these salads and you would still be consuming fewer calories than there are in one small order of french fries.

Other Picks

TENDERGRILL™ Chicken Garden Salad
with Ken's® Light Italian Dressing

360 calories
20 g fat (5 g saturated)
1,160 mg sodium

CROISSAN'WICH® Egg & Cheese

300 calories
17 g fat (6 g saturated)
740 mg sodium

Small Onion Rings

140 calories
7 g fat (1.5 g saturated)
210 mg sodium

1,000 calories
52 g fat
(10.5 g saturated)
2,040 mg sodium

Not That!

BK BIG FISH® Sandwich

with Tartar Sauce and Medium Fries

Fish is only healthy when it's not breaded and fried in partially hydrogenated oil. Here, the fry treatment translates into 7 grams of trans fats and 108 grams of carbohydrates.

WEAPON OF MASS DESTRUCTION

Triple Whopper® with Cheese and Mayo

The Impact:
1,230 calories
82 g fat (32 g saturated)
1,590 mg sodium

Hard to imagine a burger being any worse for you, unless, of course, you added bacon. (You didn't add bacon, did you?)

17

Grams of fat you save by replacing the mayo on a WHOPPER® with barbecue sauce. At 160 calories a schmear, BK's mayo is one of the worst in the fast food world.

Other Passes

600 calories
42 g fat (9 g saturated)
1,640 mg sodium

TENDERCRISP™ Chicken Garden Salad
with Ken's® Ranch Dressing

530 calories
37 g fat (12 g saturated)
1,490 mg sodium

Sausage, Egg & Cheese Biscuit

230 calories
13 g fat (3 g saturated)
380 mg sodium

Small French Fries

39

Carl's Jr.

Did You Know?

● In 1997, Carl's parent company, CKE Restaurants Inc., purchased the Southern fast food staple Hardee's. From the Six Dollar Burger™ to the smiley yellow star logo, Hardee's now borrows heavily from its West Coast brother.

HIDDEN DANGER

Breakfast

Not a single entrée item has less than 400 calories or 15 grams of fat. The 830-calorie Breakfast Burger is one of the worst breakfast sandwiches in America.

Eat This

Charbroiled BBQ Chicken™ Sandwich

360 calories
4.5 g fat
(1 g saturated)
1,150 mg sodium

Barbecue sauce and a mound of fresh produce keep the counts on this one in the safe zone.

Other Picks

Famous Star

600 calories
34 g fat (9 g saturated)
980 mg sodium

Fried Zucchini

320 calories
19 g fat (5 g saturated)
850 mg sodium

Chocolate Cake

300 calories
12 g fat (3 g saturated)
350 mg sodium

610 calories
32 g fat
(8 g saturated)
1,540 mg sodium

Not That!

Charbroiled Santa Fe Chicken™ Sandwich

By replacing the barbecue sauce with their creamy Santa Fe sauce and adding a slice of processed cheese, Carl's manages to cram an extra 27 grams of fat into this Southwest rendition.

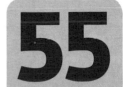

55

Grams of carbohydrates you save by wrapping a Six Dollar Burger™ in lettuce leaves

WEAPON OF MASS DESTRUCTION

The Double Six Dollar Burger™

The Impact:
1,520 calories
111 g fat
(47 g saturated)
2,760 mg sodium

Of all the gut-growing, heart-stopping, life-threatening burgers in the fast food world, there is none whose damage to your general well-being is as catastrophic as this.

Other Passes

810 calories
41 g fat (15 g saturated)
1,040 mg sodium

Super Star

410 calories
24 g fat (5 g saturated)
950 mg sodium

CrissCut® Fries

350 calories
18 g fat (7 g saturated)
330 mg sodium

Chocolate Chip Cookie

Chevy's Fresh Mex

Did You Know?

● Chevy's uses all fresh ingredients—they claim to use no cans in their kitchens. Salsas are blended every hour and tortillas are made fresh every 53 seconds during service.

LITTLE TRICK

Save 25 grams of fat by ordering the Sea Bass Grilled Tacos over the Salmon Tacos. Choose your fish wisely: The seafood at Chevy's includes the fattiest and saltiest items on the entire menu. The Shrimp Fajitas alone have 3,400 milligrams of sodium, without the tortillas!

Eat This

Santa Fe Chopped Salad
without Bacon and Cheese

338 calories
13 g fat
(2 g saturated)
247 mg sodium

Romaine lettuce is rich in vitamin E, a compound that fights the oxidative stress that ages your brain.

Other Picks

Grilled Chicken Tacos
without tamalito, rice, and cheese

595 calories
27 g fat (7 g saturated)
1,316 mg sodium

Original Famous Chicken Fajitas
without tortillas, tamalito and rice

653 calories
36 g fat (13 g saturated)
1,150 mg sodium

Black Beans
without cheese

179 calories
1 g fat (0 g saturated)
879 mg sodium

1,228 calories
77 g fat
(35 g saturated)
2,117 mg sodium

Not That!

Tostada Salad

with Chicken

The cheese alone supplies a staggering 425 calories and 36 grams of fat.

Do you really need more chips? This salad is served in a giant, sodium-packed tortilla shell.

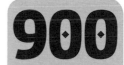

900

Number of fresh tortillas made each hour by Chevy's tortilla-making machine, El Machino. Each tortilla is served within three minutes and contains 167 calories.

GUILTY PLEASURE

Classic Sirloin

540 calories
42 g fat (14 g saturated)
820 mg sodium

If you must have a steak, this is the best choice. The sirloin has 45 fewer grams of fat than the flame-grilled rib eye, and 42 fewer than the Steak and Portobello Fajitas. The meat itself isn't necessarily the problem—less than half of the fat in a steak is saturated—it's the sauces and buttery sides that pad your gut.

Other Passes

832 calories
55 g fat (17 g saturated)
1,861 mg sodium

Grilled Fish Tacos (salmon)
without tamalito and rice

952 calories
76 g fat (24 g saturated)
3,402 mg sodium

Juicy Shrimp Fajitas
without tortillas, tamalito and rice

298 calories
15 g fat (5 mg saturated)
894 mg sodium

Refried Beans
with cheese and pico de gallo

Chick-fil-A

Did You Know?

● None of Chick-fil-A's sandwiches break the 500-calorie barrier, a rare feat in the fast food world.

● Chick-fil-A uses whole breast meat chicken in their sandwiches, Nuggets, and Chick-n-Strips®, not pressed or formed meat. The chicken arrives raw at restaurants and each piece is filleted and breaded by hand.

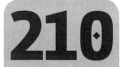

210

Calories you save by ordering chicken soup as a side instead of fries.

Eat This

Chick-fil-A® Chargrilled Chicken Sandwich

270 calories
3.5 g fat
(1 g saturated)
940 mg sodium

Instead of the mayo-slathered sandwiches you'll find at other chains, this sandwich is served with honey roasted BBQ sauce—just 60 added calories.

Other Picks

Chick-fil-A® Nuggets (8-pack)
with Barbecue Sauce

305 calories
13 g fat (2.5 g saturated)
1,020 mg sodium

Chick-fil-A® Southwest Chargrilled Salad
with Fat-Free Honey Mustard Dressing

360 calories
8 g fat (3.5 g saturated)
1,170 mg sodium

Biscuit & Gravy

330 calories
15 g fat (4 g saturated)
970 mg sodium

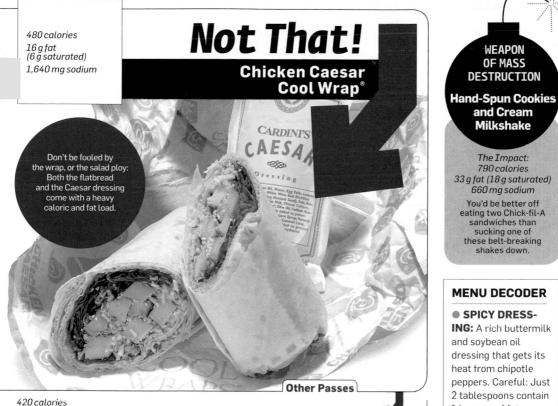

480 calories
16 g fat
(6 g saturated)
1,640 mg sodium

Not That!

Chicken Caesar Cool Wrap®

Don't be fooled by the wrap, or the salad ploy: Both the flatbread and the Caesar dressing come with a heavy caloric and fat load.

WEAPON OF MASS DESTRUCTION

Hand-Spun Cookies and Cream Milkshake

The Impact:
790 calories
33 g fat (18 g saturated)
660 mg sodium

You'd be better off eating two Chick-fil-A sandwiches than sucking one of these belt-breaking shakes down.

Other Passes

420 calories
16 g fat (3.5 g saturated)
1,300 mg sodium

Chick-fil-A® Chicken Sandwich

800 calories
60 g fat (12 g saturated)
1,745 mg sodium

Chick-fil-A® Chick-n-Strips® Salad
with Buttermilk Ranch Dressing

500 calories
20 g fat (7 g saturated)
1,260 mg sodium

Chicken, Egg & Cheese
on Sunflower Multigrain Bagel

MENU DECODER

● **SPICY DRESSING:** A rich buttermilk and soybean oil dressing that gets its heat from chipotle peppers. Careful: Just 2 tablespoons contain 14 grams of fat.

● **ICEDREAM:** Chick-fil-A's relatively low-fat take on ice cream, made with whole and nonfat milk, eggs, sugar, and corn syrup.

45

Chili's

Did You Know?

● Chili's famous a cappella rib serenade ("I want my baby back, baby back, baby back . . .") was voted the song most likely "to get stuck in your head" by *Advertising Age* magazine. With 66 grams of fat per rack, better the song in your head than the ribs in your gut.

GUILTY PLEASURE

Hot Spinach and Artichoke Dip

905 calories
36 g fat (5 g saturated)

Even if it's obscured by cheese and mayo, the 1-2 punch of artichokes and spinach brings a heap of antioxidants to Chili's healthiest starter. Still, be sure to split it.

Eat This

Sizzle & Spice Firecracker Tilapia

with Sautéed Mushrooms, Onions, and Bell Peppers, and Steamed Broccoli

470 calories
23 g fat
(5 g saturated)
1,520 mg sodium

> As long as it's not fried, this lean, moist whitefish makes a great sit-down restaurant standby.

Other Picks

Old Timer Burger®
on a Whole Wheat Bun

420 calories
27 g fat (10 g saturated)
670 mg sodium

Chicken Fajita Pita

450 calories
17 g fat (3 g saturated)
1,750 mg sodium

Dutch Apple Caramel Sweet Shot

230 calories
6 g fat (3 g saturated)
280 mg sodium

1,360 calories
73 g fat
(20 g saturated)
4,570 mg sodium

Not That!

Citrus Fire Chicken and Shrimp Fajitas

with The Works

WEAPON OF MASS DESTRUCTION

Awesome Blossom®

The Impact:
2,710 calories
203 g fat
(36 g saturated)
6,360 mg sodium
194 g carbohydrates

Easily one of the worst things you can put in your body. Avoid at all costs.

If you must have fajitas, ditch the shrimp, forget about steak completely, and stick with Classic Chicken. You'll save yourself almost 400 calories and 30 grams of fat.

MENU DECODER

● **GUILTLESS GRILL:** Like so many "healthy" menus at chain restaurants, Guiltless Grill items have less fat, but often more sugar and salt. The low-fat Black Bean Burger, for example, with 96 grams of carbohydrates, will sabotage your efforts to lose weight.

Other Passes

880 calories
51 g fat (17 g saturated)
1,190 mg sodium

Old Timer Burger®
on a Big Mouth Bun

930 calories
57 g fat (15 g saturated)
2,920 mg sodium

Smoked Turkey Sandwich

1,600 calories
78 g fat (35 g saturated)
950 mg sodium

Chocolate Chip Paradise Pie®
with Vanilla Ice Cream

Chipotle

Did You Know?

● Though we applaud Chipotle's overall drive to use fresh, natural ingredients, it doesn't always translate to better nutrition vitals: Most entrées on the menu break the dreadful 800-calorie, 40-fat-gram barrier.

LITTLE TRICK

Sub guacamole for sour cream. There may be more calories, but those come from the heart-healthy monounsaturated fats found in avocados. Plus, the guac is made fresh in-house daily.

Eat This

Chicken Burrito Bowl

with Lettuce, Black Beans, Green Tomatillo Salsa, and Sour Cream

489 calories
22 g fat
(9 g saturated)
1,006 mg sodium

Shed the rice and tortilla and you'll also shed 498 calories and 83 grams of carbohydrates.

Other Picks

Crispy Steak Tacos
with corn salsa, red tomatillo salsa, and romaine lettuce

543 calories
21 g fat (5.5 g saturated)
1,369 mg sodium

Carnitas Salad
with pinto beans, green tomatillo salsa, and cheese

495 calories
22 g fat (9 g saturated)
1,654 mg sodium

1,092 calories
44 g fat
(19 g saturated)
2,323 mg sodium

Not That!

Chicken Burrito

with Black Beans, Rice, Green
Tomatillo Salsa, Cheese, and Sour Cream

Add to
that a punishing
110 grams of
carbohydrates and the
case for avoiding
burritos at Chipotle
becomes
all too clear.

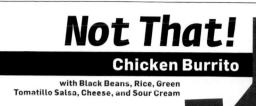

MENU DECODER

● **CHIPOTLE:** This popular burrito bar is named after a smoked jalapeño, most often found canned in a tomato-vinegar sauce called adobo. These flavor-packed, antioxidant-rich peppers are getting major play on menus across the country, but too often as a flavoring agent for fatty mayo.

● **BARBACOA:** Spicy shredded beef. The meat is first seared, then braised in liquid spiked with chipotle, garlic, and cumin until fork tender. Tasty, sure, but the least healthy meat option on the menu.

GUILTY PLEASURE

Crispy Carnitas Tacos with sour cream, lettuce, and hot salsa

560 calories,
30 g fat (11.5 g saturated)
1,426 mg sodium

The "Chef's" recommendation is actually one of the healthier meals on the menu.

788 calories
40 g fat (19 g saturated)
1,944 mg sodium

Other Passes

Barbacoa Soft Tacos

with tomato salsa, cheese,
sour cream, and romaine lettuce

858 grams
33 g fat (9 g saturated)
2,643 mg sodium

Steak Fajita Burrito

without cheese and sour cream

Cici's Pizza

Did You Know?

- It takes 20 minutes for your brain to tell your body it's full, which can be a perilous equation at free-for-all buffets like Cici's. Give your brain a head start with these three rules: Begin with a salad, never place more than two slices on your plate, and wait five minutes between finishing your plate and refueling.

- Cici's menu is 100% trans fat-free.

GUILTY PLEASURE

Apple Pizza

170 calories
4 g fat (1 g saturated)

It won't keep the doctor away, but it's a great low-impact way to satisfy your sweet tooth.

Eat This

2 Slices Olé Pizza (To-Go)

339 calories
8 g fat
(4 g saturated)
700 mg sodium

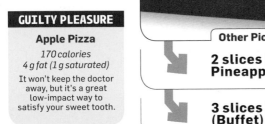

A spicy, beef-laden ode to Mexico, the Olé is the dark horse winner of the healthiest pizza on the menu.

Other Picks

2 slices Ham & Pineapple Pizza (Buffet)

282 calories
8.5 g fat (6 g saturated)
638 mg sodium

3 slices Bacon Cheddar Pizza (Buffet)

435 calories
16 g fat (6 g saturated)
937 mg sodium

446 calories
15 g fat
(11 g saturated)
1,075 mg sodium

Not That!
2 Slices Cheese Pizza (To-Go)

Don't assume the simplest slice is the best for you. Here, the bare-bones cheese pie has nearly three times the amount of saturated fat as the busy Olé.

CiCi's Pizza To·Go
CiCi's Pizza To·Go
CiCi's Pizza To·Go

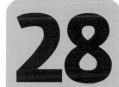

28

Percentage drop in total consumption of buffet eaters who kept their dirty dishes piled up next to them, according to a Cornell University study.

LITTLE TRICK

A slew of recent studies suggest that the size of the plate we eat on has a serious effect on our caloric intake. When at a buffet, put all of your food on a small salad plate—it will seem like you've eaten a lot more than you have, and your stomach won't know the difference.

Other Passes

350 calories
13.5 g fat (8 g saturated)
768 mg sodium

2 slices Pepperoni Pizza (Buffet)

590 calories
20 g fat (11 g saturated)
1,075 mg sodium

3 slices Sausage Pizza (Buffet)

old Stone reamery

Did You Know?

● Smoothies at Cold Stone can be made with soy milk or yogurt. Recent research has found that the calcium that accompanies dairy foods may block fat absorption and make fat less likely to be stored in the abdominal region.

LITTLE TRICK

Mix in pecans, walnuts, or almonds instead of candy—all nut mix-ins have less than 2 grams of sugar per ounce. According to a USDA study, of the 10 most popular nuts, pecans contain the most antioxidants.

Eat This

Cake Batter Light Ice Cream

with Chocolate Shavings Mix-in (6 oz. Like It™ size)

330 calories
11 g fat
(6.5 g saturated)
39 g sugars

Save 40 calories and 2 grams of fat by opting for the chocolate shavings rather than the chips.

Other Picks

Sinless Sans Fat™ Sweet Cream Ice Cream
with yellow cake, strawberries, and blueberries (6 oz)

250 calories
2.5 g fat (.5 g saturated)
23 g sugars

Chocolate Light Ice Cream
with Smucker's® Fudge mix-in in a waffle cone

480 calories
13 g fat (7.5 saturated)
54 g sugars

Raspberry Sorbet
with raspberries and Nilla® Wafers (6 oz)

270 calories
2.5 g fat (0 g saturated)
44 g sugars

Not That!

Cake Batter Ice Cream

with Cookie Dough Mix-in (6 oz. Like It™ size)

560 calories
28 g fat
(13.5 g saturated)
58 g sugars

Cookie dough adds 8 grams of fat to your dessert per hunk. Mix in Nilla® Wafers instead, for less than half the calories.

Other Passes

Our Strawberry Blonde™
Strawberry ice cream, graham cracker pie crust, strawberries, caramel, and whip topping (6 oz)

595 calories
26.5 g fat (15.5 g saturated)
57 g sugars

Dark Chocolate Ice Cream
in a dipped waffle cone

650 calories
35 g fat (22 g saturated)
60 g sugars

Raspberry Ice Cream
with graham cracker pie crust (6 oz)

520 calories
28 g fat (14.5 g saturated)
38 g sugars

MENU DECODER

● **GANACHE:** A creamy chocolate mixture used mainly as filling or frosting in Cold Stone Creamery ice cream cakes.

● **SINLESS SANS FAT™ SWEET CREAM:** A fat-free, sugar-free version of the original Sweet Cream ice cream flavor, due to nonfat milk in place of cream and maltodextrin, a cornstarch product that substitutes for sugar.

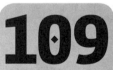

109

Times you'd have to run the length of a football field to burn off the 1,340 calories in the Gotta-Have-It™ size Chocolate Devotion™

Così

Did You Know?

● Così's menu changes 5 times a year, making adjustments for the season. Fall and winter fare tends to be heavier, with a focus on melts and dishes from the hearth, while spring and summer bring about healthier options like salads and lighter sandwiches.

2

Number of years a daily salad is estimated to increase your life span, according to LSU researchers.

Eat This

Bombay Chicken Salad

with Fat-Free Balsamic Vinaigrette and a cup of Pollo e Pasta Soup (6 oz)

294 calories
5 g fat
(2 g saturated)
1,477 mg sodium

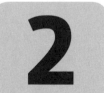

Red bell peppers have more than twice the vitamin C of green peppers and nine times the amount of vitamin A.

Skip the free flatbread that comes coupled with your salad, even if it's whole grain—both the whole grain and the original kind provide 49 grams of carbs and 740 mg of sodium. Spring for a small fruit salad instead.

Other Picks

Turkey Light sandwich

476 calories
9 g fat (0 g saturated)
1,299 mg sodium

Plain Baked Omelette Sandwich on Plain Bagel

457 calories
10 fat (3 g saturated)
333 mg sodium

Apple Tart

396 calories
6 g fat (1 g saturated)
73 mg sodium

870 calories
69 g fat
(16 g saturated)
1,242 mg sodium

Not That!

Signature Salad

with Roasted Shallot Sherry Vinaigrette and
a cup of Tomato Basil Aurora Soup (6 oz.)

One ounce
of crumbled gorgonzola
delivers 6 grams
of saturated fat.

**WEAPON
OF MASS
DESTRUCTION**

Tuna Melt

The Impact:
1,012 calories
60 g fat
1,948 mg sodium
America's worst
tuna sandwich.

MENU DECODER

● **KEFIR:** A fermented
dairy drink similar to
yogurt. Kefir contains
stomach-friendly bac-
teria that has been
shown to lower choles-
terol and enhance the
immune system.

Other Passes

772 calories
36 g fat (12 g saturated)
1,660 mg sodium

Roasted Turkey
and Brie sandwich

535 calories
21 g fat (12 g saturated)
1,001 mg sodium

Everything Bagel
with Plain Cream Cheese

960 calories
40 g fat (20 g saturated)
636 mg sodium

Cinnamon Apple Pie

GUILTY PLEASURE

S'mores for Four

(per person)
346 calories
10 g fat

Make your own s'mores
tableside for less
calories and fat than in
an oatmeal cookie.

Dairy Queen

Did You Know?

● Turning a vanilla ice cream cone into a "dipped" cone may seem like a small indulgence, but the thin crunchy coating adds 13 grams of fat to a cone.

● When in doubt, go bananas. A small Banana Split Blizzard® has 7 fewer fat grams than the small Oreo®, Cookie Dough, Peanut Butter Cup, or Strawberry CheeseQuake™ flavors, and a classic Banana Split trumps the Peanut Buster® Parfait and the Brownie Earthquake™ by at least 14 grams of fat.

Eat This

Small Chocolate Sundae

280 calories
7 g fat
(4.5 saturated)
42 g sugars

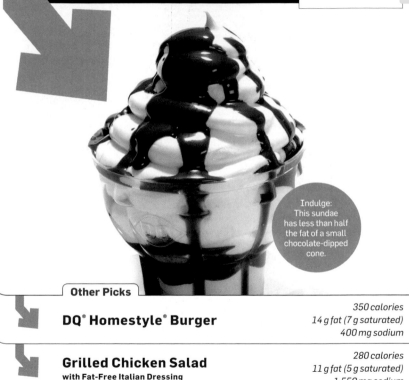

Indulge:
This sundae has less than half the fat of a small chocolate-dipped cone.

Other Picks

DQ® Homestyle® Burger
350 calories
14 g fat (7 g saturated)
400 mg sodium

Grilled Chicken Salad
with Fat-Free Italian Dressing
280 calories
11 g fat (5 g saturated)
1,550 mg sodium

DQ® Sandwich
190 calories
5 g fat (3 g saturated)
18 g sugars

720 calories
28 g fat
(14 g saturated)
78 g sugars

Not That!

Small Chocolate Chip Cookie Dough Blizzard®

Always opt for a small-sized Blizzard®—larger sizes have from .5 to 6 grams of harmful trans fat.

WEAPON OF MASS DESTRUCTION

Large Strawberry CheeseQuake™ Blizzard®

The Impact:
990 calories
39 g fat (24 g saturated)
114 g sugars

This creation combines ice cream, strawberry syrup, and hunks of cheesecake for a high-fat dairy dessert.

MENU DECODER

● **DILLY® BAR:** Introduced in 1955, the Dilly® Bar features reduced-fat ice cream dipped in chocolate for just 240 calories.

● **ARCTIC RUSH™:** A semi-frozen, slushy fruit-flavored beverage. With 48 grams of sugar in a small, it falls somewhere between soft-serve ice cream and the sugar-packed Blizzard®.

THE ORIGINAL BLIZZARD® ONLY AT DQ®

Other Passes

355 calories
33 g fat (5 g saturated)
440 mg sodium

Side Salad
with DQ® Ranch Dressing

1,270 calories
67 g fat (11 g saturated)
2,910 mg sodium

6-Piece Chicken Strip Basket™

650 calories
15 g fat (10 g saturated)
96 g sugars

Small Chocolate Malt

57

Denny's

Did You Know?

● The lights never go out at Denny's. The restaurant is open 24 hours a day, 7 days a week, 365 days a year, and serves breakfast, lunch, and dinner around the clock.

● Half of Denny's breakfast entrées contain more than 50 grams of fat, with the 1,480-calorie Smoked Sausage Scramble as the worst offender. Stick to the Fit Fare menu.

GUILTY PLEASURE

Country Fried Steak and Eggs

543 calories
34 g fat (12 g saturated)

Drop the hash browns and this hearty breakfast packs major protein for 200 calories less than the Original Grand Slam™.

Eat This

Two Fried Eggs

with Grits and Grapefruit Juice

380 calories
20 g fat
(6 g saturated)
760 mg sodium

Grapefruit juice is a great source of vitamin C and lycopene, but if you're fighting the sniffles, beware—compounds in the fruit render allergy-fighting medicines such as Allegra® nearly powerless.

With a near-perfect balance of carbs, fat, and protein, consider this Denny's real Slim Slam™.

Other Picks

Veggie-Cheese Omelette
made with Egg Beaters ®

346 calories
22 g fat (7 g saturated)
849 mg sodium

Grilled Tilapia Dinner
with rice, vegetable blend, and sliced tomatoes

603 calories
21 g fat (5.5 g saturated)
1,786 mg sodium

Vegetable Beef Soup

135 calories
4.5 g fat (1.5 g saturated)
1,290 mg sodium

890 calories
35 g fat
(9.5 g saturated)
2,673 mg sodium

Not That!

Buttermilk Pancake Platter

with Whipped Margarine and Maple Syrup

With 119 grams of carbohydrates, the pancake platter creates an early morning spike in your insulin levels, which signals your body to start storing fat.

WEAPON OF MASS DESTRUCTION

Mini Burgers with Onion Rings

The Impact:
2,220 calories
136 g fat
(31 g saturated)
3,860 mg sodium

Don't be fooled by the diminutive name: With more than a day's worth of calories and saturated fat, these minis do massive damage to your gut. In fact, 4 of Denny's 6 burgers contain more than a day's worth of fat.

Other Passes

1,480 calories
88 g fat (30 g saturated)
4,340 mg sodium

Smoked Sausage Scramble

850 calories
42 g fat (8 g saturated)
2,113 mg sodium

Fish Sandwich
with Seasoned Fries

624 calories
42 g fat (34 g saturated)
1,474 mg sodium

Clam Chowder

LITTLE TRICK

Replace your hash browns and breakfast potatoes with grits. The hot, creamy cornmeal is fat-free and will save you 118 calories.

59

Domino's

Did You Know?

● About 3 billion pizzas are sold in the U.S. each year. 400 million of those pies come from Domino's, enough for a pizza (and then some) for every man, woman, and child.

● According to the American Dairy Association, pizza is America's fourth most-craved food, behind cheese, chocolate, and ice cream.

LITTLE TRICK

Substitute cheddar cheese on your next 'za. It might make an Italian shudder, but Domino's cheddar has a third of the calories and fat of mozzarella.

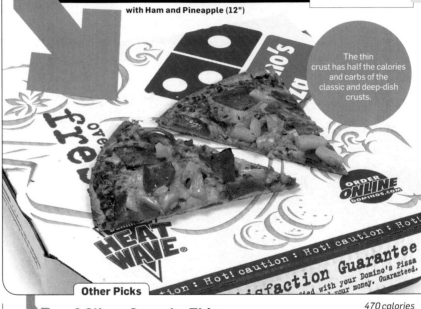

Eat This

2 Slices Crunchy Thin Crust Pizza

with Ham and Pineapple (12")

300 calories
16 g fat
(4 g saturated)
630 mg sodium

The thin crust has half the calories and carbs of the classic and deep-dish crusts.

ORDER ONLINE DOMINOS.COM

Other Picks

2 Slices Crunchy Thin Crust Deluxe Feast® (12")

470 calories
32 g fat (12 g saturated)
1,240 mg sodium

Grilled Chicken Caesar
with Light Italian Dressing

220 calories
5.5 g fat (2 g saturated)
1,400 mg sodium

Six Buffalo Chicken Kickers™
with Hot Dipping Cup

390 calories
21 g fat (4 g saturated)
1,060 mg sodium

510 calories
22 g fat
(8 g saturated)
950 mg sodium

Not That!

2 Slices Classic Hand-Tossed Pizza

with Pepperoni (12")

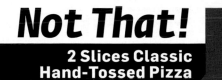

Heavy on sodium and fat, pepperoni is one of the worst things you can put on a pizza.

WEAPON OF MASS DESTRUCTION

Cheesy Bread with Garlic Dipping Sauce

The Impact:
1,560 calories
105 g fat
(28 g saturated fat)
1,510 mg sodium

You're better off eating an entire medium thin-crust pizza.

MENU DECODER

● **PHILLY CHEESE STEAK:** A pizza loaded with slices of steak, Provolone, onions, green peppers, mushrooms, and American cheese, with 14 grams of fat in 2 slices (12")

● **GARLIC DIPPING SAUCE:** Partially hydrogenated soybean oil with "natural garlic flavor." With 7 grams of trans fats in each tiny tub, dip at your own demise.

Other Passes

780 calories
47 g fat (17 g saturated)
2,230 mg sodium

2 Slices Ultimate Deep Dish ExtravaganZZa Feast® (12")

370 calories
32 g fat (10 g saturated)
610 mg sodium

Garden Fresh Salad
with Blue Cheese Dressing

840 calories
64 g fat (15 g saturated)
1,710 mg sodium

Six Hot Buffalo Wings
with Blue Cheese Dipping Cup

Dunkin' Donuts

Did You Know?

● Drinking four 6-ounce cups of caffeinated coffee a day reduces your risk of dying of heart disease by 53 percent, say researchers at Brooklyn College. The study tracked the caffeine intakes of 6,500 people for 2 years.

WEAPON OF MASS DESTRUCTION

Peanut Butter Cup Cookie

The Impact:
590 calories
29 g fat (13 g saturated)
73 g carbohydrates

This cookie is worse than 10 Oreos®.

Eat This

Ham Egg & Cheese English Muffin Sandwich

310 calories
10 g fat
(5 g saturated)
1,270 mg sodium

English muffins have a fraction of the carbohydrates of a bagel, and none of the trans fats of the donuts and croissants.

Other Picks

Glazed Donut	180 calories 8 g fat (1.5 g saturated) 12 g sugars
Ham and Swiss Sandwich	360 calories 11 g fat (5 g saturated) 1,120 mg sodium
Hot Latte Lite	70 calories 0 g fat 9 g sugars

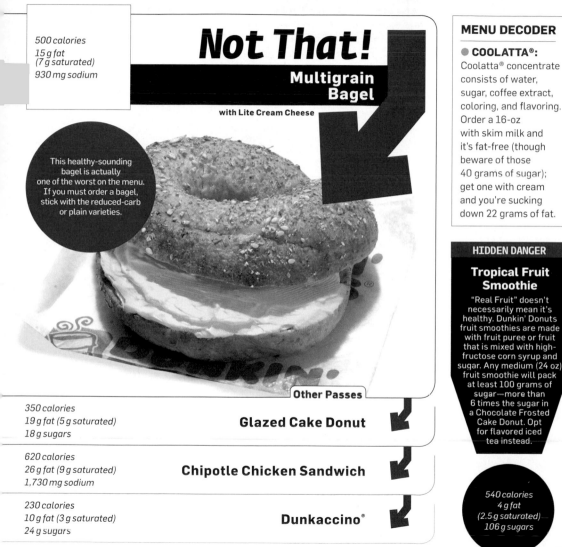

500 calories
15 g fat
(7 g saturated)
930 mg sodium

Not That!

Multigrain Bagel

with Lite Cream Cheese

This healthy-sounding bagel is actually one of the worst on the menu. If you must order a bagel, stick with the reduced-carb or plain varieties.

Other Passes

350 calories
19 g fat (5 g saturated)
18 g sugars

Glazed Cake Donut

620 calories
26 g fat (9 g saturated)
1,730 mg sodium

Chipotle Chicken Sandwich

230 calories
10 g fat (3 g saturated)
24 g sugars

Dunkaccino®

MENU DECODER

● **COOLATTA®:**
Coolatta® concentrate consists of water, sugar, coffee extract, coloring, and flavoring. Order a 16-oz with skim milk and it's fat-free (though beware of those 40 grams of sugar); get one with cream and you're sucking down 22 grams of fat.

HIDDEN DANGER

Tropical Fruit Smoothie

"Real Fruit" doesn't necessarily mean it's healthy. Dunkin' Donuts fruit smoothies are made with fruit puree or fruit that is mixed with high-fructose corn syrup and sugar. Any medium (24 oz) fruit smoothie will pack at least 100 grams of sugar—more than 6 times the sugar in a Chocolate Frosted Cake Donut. Opt for flavored iced tea instead.

540 calories
4 g fat
(2.5 g saturated)
106 g sugars

Einstein Bros/Noah's

Did You Know?

● These bagel titans are owned by the New World Restaurant Group and have nearly identical menus.

GUILTY PLEASURE

Butternut Squash Soup (bowl)

380 calories
23 g fat (14 g saturated)
1,500 mg sodium

The fat maybe slightly excessive, but it also helps your body better absorb the heavy hit of cancer-fighting carotenoids provided by the squash.

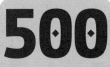

500

Dollars, in millions, that Americans spend on bagels each year.

Eat This

Albacore Tuna Salad Sandwich
on Wheat

465 calories
16.5 g fat
(2 g saturated)
470 mg sodium

Albacore tuna is rich in omega-3s, which help maintain your brain's processing speed.

Other Picks

Egg Frittata

430 calories
10 g fat (3 g saturated)
690 mg sodium

Chicken Portabello Sesame Bagel Dog

480 calories
23 g fat (12 g saturated)
1,240 mg sodium

Café Latte (Hot)
(12 oz)

140 calories
5 g fat (3.5 g saturated)
13 g sugars

530 calories
21 g fat
(7 g saturated)
1,670 mg sodium

Not That!

Albacore Tuna Panini Melt

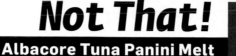

The Swiss-mozzarella-mayo combo ratchets up the fat, while the large ciabatta roll contributes heavily to the panini's 51 grams of carbs.

Other Passes

500 calories
24 g fat (13 g fat)
690 mg sodium

Veg-Out® Sandwich
on Sesame Seed Bagel

660 calories
27 g fat (19 g saturated)
1,150 mg sodium

Lox & Bagel

460 calories
18 g fat (14 g saturated)
50 g sugars

Café Latte (Frozen)
(18 oz)

LITTLE TRICK

Try substituting hummus for mayonnaise in sandwiches, or for cream cheese on bagels: Beyond being lower in fat and calories than both, this smooth spread of pureed chickpeas and tahini adds a dose of protein and fiber to anything it touches.

MENU DECODER

● **CHALLAH:**
A yeasty, egg-enriched bread traditionally eaten on many Jewish holidays. Because of its richness, challah is often used to make French toast. Einstein Bros' version, however, is fairly light on the eggs, which makes it a reasonable choice for sandwiches.

Fazoli's

● In 2007, Fazoli's revamped their menu offerings with the Aaaahtalian menu, touting more than 50 items with zero grams trans fat. Trans-fat holdouts include the ziti with meat sauce, pizza, and most baked pasta dishes.

HIDDEN DANGER

Breadsticks

At 450 calories and 21 grams of fat for 3 breadsticks, the all-you-can-eat policy can do major damage before the meal even begins.

Eat This

Small Penne with Marinara

and Garlic Shrimp and Garden Side Salad with Fat-Free Italian

660 calories
14.5 g fat
(2.5 g saturated)
1,985 mg sodium

Even though this dish is low in fat, don't let it become a staple of your diet: With 93 grams of carbohydrates, it can still do damage to your waistline.

Other Picks

Cheese Slice and Garden Side Salad
with Fat-Free Italian Dressing

320 calories
11 g fat (4 g saturated)
1,105 mg sodium

Grilled Chicken Panini

540 calories
18 g fat (4.5 g saturated)
1,360 mg sodium

Chicken and Fruit Salad
with Fat-Free Honey Mustard

280 calories
1.5 g fat (0 g saturated)
1,050 mg sodium

Not That!

Spaghetti with Marinara

and Spicy Italian Sausage and Caesar Side Salad

1,030 calories
53.5 g fat
(12 g saturated)
2,040 mg sodium

The Italian sausage alone adds 21 grams of fat. Want meat with your pasta? Stick with the lean, peppery chicken.

Other Passes

Baked Spaghetti
with Meatballs

940 calories
40 g fat (17 g saturated)
2,370 mg sodium

Original Submarino®

940 calories
58 g fat (17 g saturated)
3,040 mg sodium

Parmesan Chicken Salad
with Ranch Dressing

580 calories
39 g fat (8.5 g saturated)
1,270 mg sodium

MENU DECODER

● **PIZZA SAUCE:** Fazoli's pizza sauce contains an unexpected ingredient—carrot puree—adding a hint of natural sweetness to the usual suspects: tomato puree, diced tomatoes, sugar, olive oil, garlic, and spices. Carrots contain vitamin E and carotenoids, which help your skin resist UV damage.

● **LEMON ICE:** Lemon "flavoring" and high-fructose corn syrup. A large contains 72 grams of sugar.

GUILTY PLEASURE

Meat Lasagna

510 calories
25 g fat

Considering that it's a tower of noodles, beef, and cheese, the lasagna strikes a surprisingly decent balance of protein, fat, and carbohydrates, making it the best of the baked pasta dishes.

Five Guys Burgers and

Did You Know?

● As of October 2007, there were 1,000 new Five Guys in the building or planning stage, making it one of the fastest-growing chains in the U.S.

● Like the West Coast staple, In-N-Out, Five Guys offers only a few options for its customers: burgers, fries, and hot dogs.

GUILTY PLEASURE

Bacon
(2 slices)

80 calories
7 g fat (3 g saturated)
260 mg sodium

If you're looking to indulge, skip the American cheese and reward yourself with a few slices of bacon—it has less saturated fat and sodium.

Eat This

Little Hamburger

with Sautéed Mushrooms, Onions, Jalapeños and A1® Steak Sauce

578 calories
28 g fat
(11.5 g saturated)
995 mg sodium

Embrace the heat: Eating peppers can help you lose weight, fight colds, and even avoid ulcers.

With just 15 calories, zero fat, and a whole lot more flavor, A1® makes the perfect alternative to mayo.

Other Picks

Little Hamburger
with onions, lettuce, tomato, ketchup, and pickles

583 calories
28 g fat (11.5 g saturated)
892 mg sodium

BLT: 4 slices of bacon, lettuce, tomato, and mustard

434 calories
23 g fat (9.5 g saturated)
915 mg sodium

Fries

735 calories
45 g fat
(17 g saturated)
1,011 mg sodium

Not That!

Little Cheeseburger

with Lettuce, Tomato, Mayo, and Ketchup

There are 6 grams of fat in just one slice of Kraft® American cheese.

WEAPON OF MASS DESTRUCTION

Bacon Cheeseburger
with barbecue sauce and mayo with regular fries

The Impact:
1,750 calories
82 g fat (26 g saturated)
1,565 mg sodium

The combination of cheese, bacon, and mayo stacks up saturated fat, and the regular-sized fries piles on 78 grams of carbohydrates.

LITTLE TRICK

A regular hamburger or cheeseburger at Five Guys means two beef patties. Order the "little" burger with one patty, then load up on vegetables like mushrooms, peppers, onions, tomatoes, and lettuce— veggie add-ons are free at Five Guys.

Other Passes

585 calories
35 g fat (15.5 g saturated)
1,461 mg sodium

Hot Dog

with ketchup, mustard, onions, and relish

815 calories
52 g fat (20 g saturated)
1,356 mg sodium

Little Cheeseburger

with bacon, onions, steak sauce, and mayo

Häagen-Dazs

Did You Know?

● Häagen-Dazs is not Scandinavian, as is commonly believed; it is simply two made-up words meant to appear Scandinavian to Americans.

LITTLE TRICK

Opt for frozen yogurt instead of fruit sorbet: The fruit sorbets have about 50 percent more sugar than the yogurt.

GUILTY PLEASURE

Pomegranate Chip Ice Cream (¹/₂ cup)

*280 calories
16 g fat (10 g saturated)
28 g sugars*

It may be high in fat, but the pomegranate that flavors this is loaded with heart-healthy polyphenols, and has been proven to increase blood flow to the heart by up to 17 percent.

Eat This

Zesty Lemon Sorbet

(¹/₂ cup)

*110 calories
0 g fat
29 g sugars*

Sugar, lemon juice concentrate, and fruit pectin flavor this fat-free indulgence. Although sorbet can be high in sugar, it has less than half the calories of ice cream.

Other Picks

Dulce de Leche Frozen Yogurt
(¹/₂ cup)

*190 calories
2.5 g fat (2 g saturated)
25 g sugars*

Vanilla Raspberry Swirl Frozen Yogurt
(¹/₂ cup)

*170 calories
2.5 fat (1.5 g saturated)
24 g sugars*

Not That!
Mango Ice Cream
(½ cup)

250 calories
14 g fat
(8 g saturated)
27 g sugars

Opt for the mango sorbet instead of the ice cream for fat-free mango flavor.

gen-Dazs®

5

Number of ingredients in Häagen-Dazs's vanilla, chocolate, strawberry, and coffee ice creams.

MENU DECODER

● **SUPER PREMIUM:** Unlike soft serve ice cream, Häagen-Dazs is very dense, with little air mixed in during production and no emulsifiers used. The label also indicates high butterfat content.

● **MAYAN CHOCOLATE:** The word "chocolate" comes from the Maya word *xocoatl*, which means "bitter water." But this chocolate creation is flavored with Dutched chocolate, brown sugar, cinnamon, and cinnamon extract.

Other Passes

Vanilla Caramel Brownie Light Ice Cream
(½ cup)

240 calories
7 g fat (4 g saturated)
31 g sugars

Black Raspberry Chip Ice Cream
(½ cup)

280 calories
18 g fat (11 g saturated)
24 g sugars

Hardee's

Did You Know?

● Hardee's employees make biscuits from scratch every morning on location. But like any good biscuit, these come at a steep price: 370 calories and 23 grams of fat: more than in a cheeseburger from the lunch menu.

HIDDEN DANGER

Country Breakfast Burrito

The most destructive handheld breakfast in America. According to Hardee's marketing chief, "This is really designed to fill you up." More like fill you out.

920 calories
60 g fat
(23 g saturated)
1,970 mg sodium

Eat This

⅓ lb Low Carb Thickburger

420 calories
32 g fat
(12 g saturated)
1,010 mg sodium

By shedding the bun in favor of a lettuce wrap, you cut the calories and fat in half.

Other Picks

Charbroiled BBQ Chicken Sandwich

415 calories
5 g fat (1 g saturated)
1,175 mg sodium

Sunrise Croissant

210 calories
10 g fat (4 g saturated)
200 mg sodium

Mashed Potatoes and Gravy

110 calories
3 g fat (0 g saturated)
630 mg sodium

850 calories
57 g fat
(22 g saturated)
1,470 mg sodium

Not That!

⅓ lb Thickburger

WEAPON OF MASS DESTRUCTION

⅔ lb Monster Thickburger

The Impact:
1,420 calories
108 g fat
(43 g saturated)
2,770 mg sodium
230 mg cholesterol

More sodium and fat than you should get in a day, and more saturated fat than you want in two.

Can't do the lettuce thing? Then downsize to a double hamburger—it has half the calories and a third of the fat.

MENU DECODER

● **COUNTRY HAM:** Southern-style cured ham, similar to an Italian prosciutto, often eaten on biscuits for breakfast. Because it's cured in salt and nitrates, even a small piece of country ham can launch a dish's sodium count into the stratosphere.

Other Passes

770 calories
36 g fat (8 g saturated)
2,000 mg sodium

Big Chicken Fillet Sandwich

560 calories
38 g fat (11 g saturated)
1,360 mg sodium

Bacon, Egg & Cheese Biscuit

390 calories
19 g fat (4 g saturated)
240 mg sodium

Small French Fries

In-N-Out Burger

Did You Know?

● In-N-Out has a cult following primarily from their standards for freshness. They do not own a freezer, microwave, or heat lamp. They peel and cut fries from whole potatoes on site. And they butcher, grind, and ship all their own beef.

WEAPON OF MASS DESTRUCTION

Chocolate Shake

690 calories
55 g fat (24 g saturated)

It might be made with real ice cream, but it still has as much saturated fat as six burgers.

Eat This

Double-Double® Hamburger Protein® Style

with Grilled Onions, Tomatoes, Mustard, and Ketchup

350 calories
22 g fat
(11 g saturated)
960 mg sodium

Order any burger on the menu "protein style" and they'll dispose of the bun and wrap the patties in lettuce instead. The savings is huge: 150 calories and 30 grams of carbohydrates.

Other Picks

Hamburger
with onion, tomato, lettuce, and ketchup

310 calories
10 g fat (4 g saturated)
730 mg sodium

Cheeseburger

480 calories
27 g fat (10 g saturated)
1,000 mg sodium

16 oz Arnold Palmer
(Half lemonade, half iced tea)

90 calories
0 g fat
19 g sugars

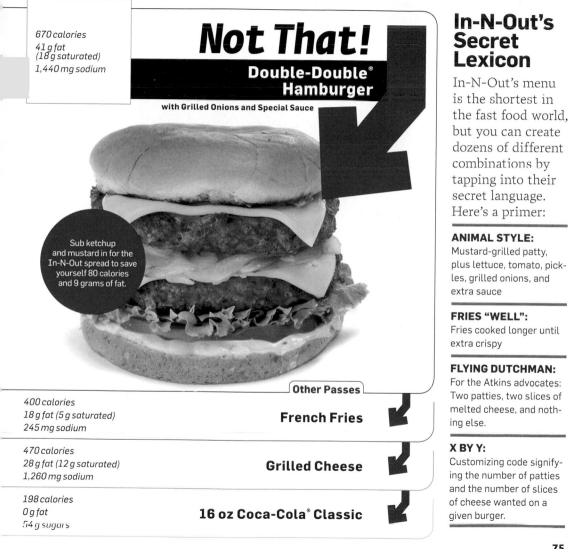

670 calories
41 g fat
(18 g saturated)
1,440 mg sodium

Not That!

Double-Double® Hamburger

with Grilled Onions and Special Sauce

Sub ketchup and mustard in for the In-N-Out spread to save yourself 80 calories and 9 grams of fat.

Other Passes

400 calories
18 g fat (5 g saturated)
245 mg sodium

French Fries

470 calories
28 g fat (12 g saturated)
1,260 mg sodium

Grilled Cheese

198 calories
0 g fat
54 g sugars

16 oz Coca-Cola® Classic

In-N-Out's Secret Lexicon

In-N-Out's menu is the shortest in the fast food world, but you can create dozens of different combinations by tapping into their secret language. Here's a primer:

ANIMAL STYLE: Mustard-grilled patty, plus lettuce, tomato, pickles, grilled onions, and extra sauce

FRIES "WELL": Fries cooked longer until extra crispy

FLYING DUTCHMAN: For the Atkins advocates: Two patties, two slices of melted cheese, and nothing else.

X BY Y: Customizing code signifying the number of patties and the number of slices of cheese wanted on a given burger.

Jack in the Box

Did You Know?

● Unlike many other fast food restaurants that have made the shift away from trans fats, Jack in the Box's menu has a number of items with more than 5 grams of the stuff. Avoid the brunt of it by staying away from anything that touches the deep fryer.

LITTLE TRICK

Try a Regular Beef Taco instead of a small fries with your next combo meal. Sound crazy? Here's what you'll save: 180 calories, 9 grams of fat, 4 grams of trans fats, and 26 grams of carbohydrates.

Eat This

Chicken Fajita Pita

and Side Salad with Fire Roasted Salsa

335 calories
12 g fat
(5 g saturated)
1,275 mg sodium

Try dressing your salads with Jack's Fire Roasted Salsa: It'll cost you exactly 5 calories.

Loaded with fresh veggies in a fairly harmless pita vessel, this is the healthiest entrée available at Jack's, hands down.

Other Picks

Asian Grilled Chicken Salad
with Roasted Slivered Almonds
and Low-Fat Balsamic Dressing

310 calories
12.5 g fat (0.5 g saturated)
1,085 mg sodium

Hamburger Deluxe
with Ketchup and Mustard
(hold the Mayo-Onion Sauce)

280 calories
11 g fat (5.5 g saturated)
475 mg sodium

Breakfast Jack®

290 calories
12 g fat (4.5 g saturated)
760 mg sodium

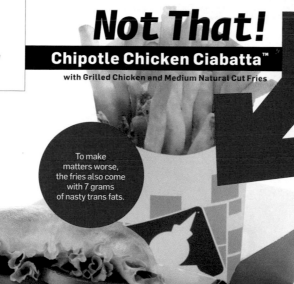

1,140 calories
51 g fat
(14 g saturated)
3,000 mg sodium

Not That!

Chipotle Chicken Ciabatta™

with Grilled Chicken and Medium Natural Cut Fries

To make matters worse, the fries also come with 7 grams of nasty trans fats.

GUILTY PLEASURE

Bacon Breakfast Jack

300 calories
14 g fat (5 g saturated)
730 mg sodium

16 grams of protein makes this a surprisingly good way to start your day. But skip breakfast burritos and biscuits at all costs.

SAUCE DECODER

● **MAYO-ONION SAUCE:** Soybean oil, egg yolks, high-fructose corn syrup, onion powder. 90 calories, 10 g of fat.

● **BARBECUE DIPPING SAUCE:** Vinegar, tomato paste, brown sugar, high-fructose corn syrup, molasses, spices. 45 calories, 0 g fat.

● **FIRE ROASTED TOMATO SALSA:** Tomato, roasted tomato puree, onions, jalapeños, cilantro. 5 calories, 0 g fat.

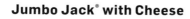

Other Passes

590 calories
39 g fat (10.5 g saturated)
1,820 mg sodium

Southwest Chicken Salad
with Grilled Chicken and Creamy Southwest Dressing

690 calories
42 g fat (16 g saturated)
1,310 mg sodium

Jumbo Jack® with Cheese

740 calories
55 g fat (17 g saturated)
1,430 mg sodium

Sausage, Egg & Cheese Biscuit

Jamba Juice

Did You Know?

● There are 5 servings of fruit in each of the all-fruit smoothies at Jamba Juice (Original size). Tacking on a "vita boost" gives you 100 percent of your daily value of 21 different vitamins and minerals, including calcium and vitamins A, C, D, E, and K.

HIDDEN DANGER

Aloha Pineapple (30 oz)

More sugar than a banana split at Baskin-Robbins®!

650 calories
142 g sugars

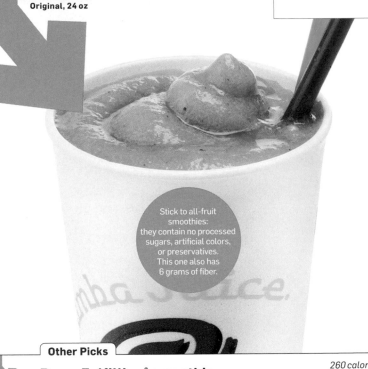

Eat This

Peach Perfection™ Smoothie
Original, 24 oz

320 calories
0.5 g fat
(0 g saturated)
78 g carbohydrates

Stick to all-fruit smoothies: they contain no processed sugars, artificial colors, or preservatives. This one also has 6 grams of fiber.

Other Picks

Berry Fulfilling® smoothie
Original, 24 oz

260 calories
1 g fat (0 g saturated)
57 g carbohydrates

Cheddar Jalapeño Twist

250 calories
5 g fat (2.5 g saturated)
540 mg sodium

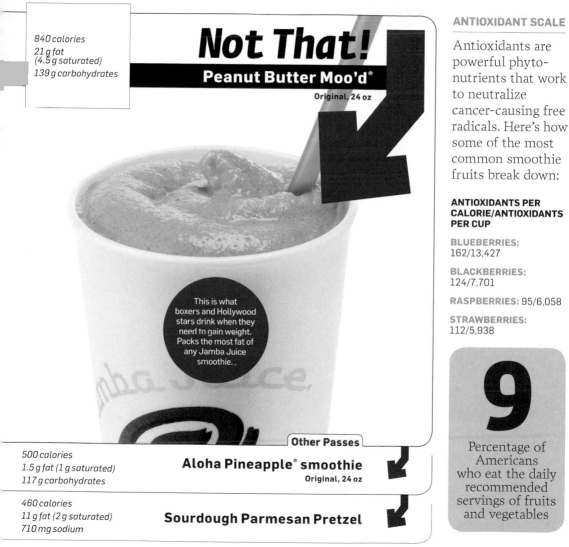

840 calories
21 g fat
(4.5 g saturated)
139 g carbohydrates

Not That!

Peanut Butter Moo'd®

Original, 24 oz

This is what boxers and Hollywood stars drink when they need to gain weight. Packs the most fat of any Jamba Juice smoothie.

Other Passes

500 calories
1.5 g fat (1 g saturated)
117 g carbohydrates

Aloha Pineapple® smoothie
Original, 24 oz

460 calories
11 g fat (2 g saturated)
710 mg sodium

Sourdough Parmesan Pretzel

ANTIOXIDANT SCALE

Antioxidants are powerful phyto-nutrients that work to neutralize cancer-causing free radicals. Here's how some of the most common smoothie fruits break down:

ANTIOXIDANTS PER CALORIE/ANTIOXIDANTS PER CUP

BLUEBERRIES:
162/13,427

BLACKBERRIES:
124/7,701

RASPBERRIES: 95/6,058

STRAWBERRIES:
112/5,938

9

Percentage of Americans who eat the daily recommended servings of fruits and vegetables

Jimmy John's

Did You Know?

● Jimmy John's vegetables are from local sources and delivered on a daily basis. Unlike at Subway, nothing is delivered pre-sliced. Meat and vegetables are cut fresh in-house every day.

● To maintain a focus on high-quality sandwiches, Jimmy John's franchises are not allowed to sell salads or soup.

LITTLE TRICK

Substitute avocado spread for mayo and knock off 200 calories, 24 grams of fat, and 98 grams of sodium.

Eat This

Turkey Breast Slim Sub

with Alfalfa Sprouts, Tomatoes, Onion, Cucumber, and Avocado Spread

426 calories
2 g fat
(1 g saturated)
1,439 mg sodium

Start with a Plain Slim and build a healthier sandwich by subbing vegetables for cheese, mayo, and dressings.

Other Picks

Totally Tuna™ sub

507 calories
20 g fat (3.5 g saturated)
1,279 mg sodium

Vegetarian sub
Avocado spread, cucumber, lettuce, tomatoes, alfalfa sprouts

290 calories
1.5 g fat (1 g saturated)
628 mg sodium

Not That!

Turkey Tom®

with Alfalfa Sprouts, Tomatoes, Lettuce, and Mayo

555 calories
26 g fat
(4 g saturated)
1,342 mg sodium

Jimmy John's is liberal with the mayo—Hellmann's® alone adds 25 grams of fat to your lunch. Stick with mustard and win back all 25 grams.

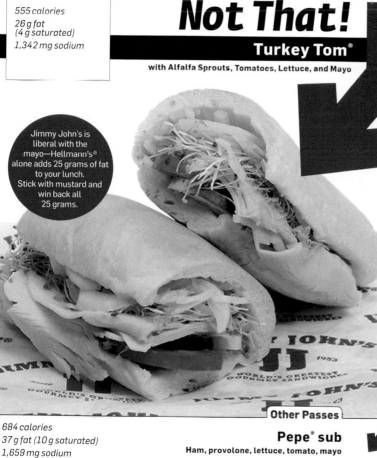

WEAPON OF MASS DESTRUCTION

The J.J. Gargantuan™

The Impact:
1,008 calories
55 g fat (15 g saturated)
3,783 mg sodium

A vegetarian's nightmare invented by Jimmy John's heavy-handed brother, Huey. This gut bomb features Genoa salami, smoked ham, capicola, roast beef, smoked turkey, and provolone smothered with mayo and Italian dressing.

MENU DECODER

● **PLAIN SLIMS:** Any Jimmy John's sub sandwich, minus the vegetables and the sauce.

● **UNWICH:** A Jimmy John's sandwich served in a lettuce wrap instead of bread. You can request any sandwich as an Unwich.

Other Passes

Pepe® sub
Ham, provolone, lettuce, tomato, mayo

684 calories
37 g fat (10 g saturated)
1,659 mg sodium

Gourmet Veggie Club®
Provolone, avocado, cucumber, alfalfa sprouts, lettuce, tomato, mayo

856 calories
46 g fat (15 g saturated)
1,500 mg sodium

81

KFC

Did You Know?

● Kentucky Fried Chicken abbreviated its name in 1991. Some speculate the Colonel made the switch to deemphasize the fact that most of the food on the menu is fried.

● KFC products are the most popularly requested items for death row inmates' last meals.

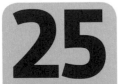

25

Grams of fat saved when you toss a Caesar salad with fat-free ranch instead of the hazardous Creamy Parmesan dressing

Eat This

3 Crispy Strips

Green Beans and 3" Corn on the Cob

470 calories
22 g fat
(4 g saturated)
1,775 mg sodium

Order a side of green beans for a good source of vitamins K, A, and C— key vitamins in maintaining strong bones and reducing cancer-causing free radicals.

Other Picks

Honey BBQ KFC Snacker®

210 calories
3 g fat (.5 g saturated)
530 mg sodium

Roasted BLT Salad
with Fat Free Hidden Valley ® Ranch Dressing

235 calories
6 g fat (2 g saturated)
1,290 mg sodium

Sweet Life Oatmeal Raisin Cookie

150 calories
5 g fat (2.5 g saturated)
135 mg sodium

740 calories
35 g fat
(9 g saturated)
2,350 mg sodium

Not That!

KFC Famous Bowl™

Mashed Potato with Gravy

Beyond the sky-high sodium, the starchy mound within contains 80 grams of carbohydrates.

GUILTY PLEASURE

Mashed Potatoes and Gravy

140 calories
5 g fat (1 g saturated)
560 mg sodium

Not the fatty carb bomb that mashed potatoes can be at other establishments. Choose this over potato wedges and save 110 calories.

MENU DECODER

● **SECRET RECIPE®:** 11-ingredient herb and spice mix concocted by the Colonel himself back in the 1930s. With his handwritten recipe locked in a safe somewhere in Louisville, Kentucky, KFC claims that two separate companies contribute distinct parts of the recipe, ensuring that only a select few people actually know all 11 ingredients. True or not, the Colonel's Original Recipe® has become a powerful marketing angle for KFC over the years.

Other Passes

400 calories
26 g fat (4.5 g saturated)
1,160 mg sodium

Popcorn Chicken—Individual

670 calories
48 g fat (11 g saturated)
1,755 mg sodium

Crispy Caesar Salad
with Creamy Parmesan Caesar Dressing and Croutons

370 calories
20 g fat (6 g saturated)
260 mg sodium

Apple Pie Minis (3)

Krispy Kreme

Did You Know?

● Free-standing Krispy Kreme restaurants have neon signs that light up "HOT DOUGHNUTS NOW" when fresh doughnuts are rolling off the production line.

● Every doughnut on Krispy Kreme's menu has at least 3.5 grams of trans fats. The worst? The apple fritter, with 7 grams of the bad stuff.

LITTLE TRICK

Avoid any doughnut with "Kreme" in the name: They are the only doughnuts to roll out 20+ grams of fat each.

Eat This

Whole Wheat Glazed Doughnut

180 calories
11 g fat
(3 g saturated)
10 g sugars

The only doughnut with fiber, this provides 2 grams' worth.

With only 19 grams of carbohydrates, the whole wheat clocks in at less than half of the opponent's—and nearly every other doughnut on the menu.

Other Picks

Original Glazed Doughnut Holes
(5 pieces)

200 calories
11 g fat (2.5 g saturated)
15 g sugars

Very Berry Chiller
(12 oz, without whipped cream)

170 calories
0 g fat
43 g sugars

330 calories
17 g fat
(4 g saturated)
28 g sugars

Not That!

Glazed Blueberry Cake Doughnut

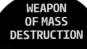

WEAPON OF MASS DESTRUCTION

20 oz Chocolate, Chocolate Chiller

1,050 calories
42 g fat (36 g saturated)
100 g sugars

In a few foul sips, you'll soak up half your day's calorie allotment, and nearly twice the amount of saturated fat that you're supposed to ingest.

Don't be fooled by the fruit in the name: Those little flecks of blue can't reverse the impact of 28 grams of sugar.

MENU DECODER

● **DULCE DE LECHE:** Latin America's answer to caramel, used as a filling in a variety of desserts from Mexico to Argentina. The common recipe calls for slow-boiled sweetened condensed milk. Krispy Kreme's sticky spin-off, the Dulce De Leche doughnut, has 18 grams of fat.

Other Passes

380 calories
21 g fat (5 g saturated)
26 g sugars

Caramel Kreme Crunch

670 calories
28 g fat (24 g saturated)
58 g sugars

Mocha Dream Chiller
(12 oz)

85

Little Caesars

Did You Know?

● "Little Caesar" was the nickname that chain founder Marian Ilitch called her husband, Mike. The pair first set up shop in a strip mall in the suburbs of Detroit.

● 1.5 ounces of Little Caesars® Italian, ranch, Greek, and Caesar salad dressings have at least 7 more grams of fat than any slice of pizza on the menu.

GUILTY PLEASURE

Hawaiian Pizza
(2 slices, thin crust)

172 calories
15 g fat (7 g saturated)

Ham and pineapple add a meager 12 calories and virtually no fat to a slice, plus provide a hit of protein and bromelain, a natural anti-inflammatory found in pineapple.

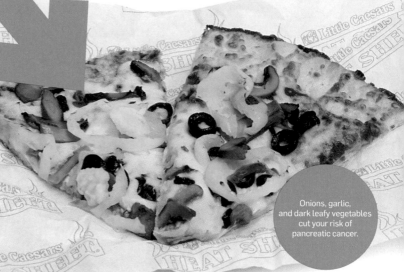

Eat This

One slice Veggie Pizza (14")
with a Tossed Salad with Fat-Free Italian Dressing (6.2 oz)

365 calories
11 g fat
(4.5 g saturated)
1,270 mg sodium

Onions, garlic, and dark leafy vegetables cut your risk of pancreatic cancer.

Other Picks

Two sticks Cinnamon Crazy Bread®

100 calories
2 g fat (0 g saturated)
95 mg sodium

One slice Thin Crust Cheese Pizza
with Ham topping (12")

145 calories
7 g fat (3 g saturated)
245 mg sodium

Two slices Cheese Pizza (12")

360 calories
12 g fat (6 g saturated)
580 mg sodium

670 calories
48.5 g fat
(15.5 g saturated)
1,420 g sodium

Not That!

One slice Meatsa Pizza (14")

with a Greek Salad with Greek dressing (9.5 oz)

29 grams of fat in the Greek dressing all but cancel out the veggies' health benefits

LITTLE TRICK

Crazy Bread® can be ordered without the Parmesan cheese topping and pizza can be ordered with half the usual amount of cheese to cut back heavily on fat. Order pizza with half the cheese and extra sauce for a dose of lycopene—an antioxidant that fights prostate cancer and protects your skin from UV damage.

Other Passes

130 calories
6 g fat (2.5 g saturated)
310 mg sodium

Two pieces Italian Cheese Bread®

640 calories
29 g fat (3 g saturated)
1,540 mg sodium

Ham & Cheese Deli Sandwich

460 calories
18 g fat (8 g saturated)
680 mg sodium

Two slices Deep Dish Cheese Pizza

(medium)

MENU DECODER

● **CRAZY BREAD®:**
Pizza dough that has been brushed with garlic butter and topped with Parmesan cheese.

● **BABY PAN!PAN!®:**
A square, individual-sized deep dish pizza topped with cheese and pepperoni, packing 16 grams of fat and 630 mg of sodium.

Long John Silver's

Did You Know?

● Long John Silver's battered fish sandwiches are made of Alaskan pollock, hoki, or hake, depending on the location. Alaskan pollock is the largest source of food fish in the world, most coming from the Bering Sea.

● Long John Silver's signature battered fish and shrimp are fried in partially hydrogenated soybean oil, which contains unhealthy omega-6 fats. According to health experts, the average American now eats 10 to 20 times as much omega-6 fat as heart-healthy omega-3 fats.

Eat This

Baked Cod (2 pieces)
with a Corn Cobette

340 calories
11 g fat
(2.5 g saturated)
470 mg sodium

Chow down 46 grams of protein with the baked cod, plus a shot of heart-healthy fat.

Dig in with a fork instead of ordering a sandwich—Long John Silver's buns contain high-fructose corn syrup and partially hydrogenated oils.

Other Picks

Chicken Sandwich

360 calories
15 g fat (3.5 g saturated)
900 mg sodium

Battered Shrimp (3 pieces)

135 calories
9 g fat (3 g saturated)
480 mg sodium

Pineapple Cream Pie

290 calories
13 g fat (7 g saturated)

HIDDEN DANGER

Crispy Chicken Club Salad with Ranch

The nutritional equivalent of fish and chips. Order the Shrimp and Seafood Salad with Lite Italian and save 460 calories.

750 calories
42 g fat
(10.5 g saturated)
1,930 mg sodium

Not That!

Battered Fish (2 pieces)

with Small French Fries

If you must dip, choose cocktail sauce rather than tartar sauce to cut 75 calories and 9 grams of fat.

740 calories
54 g fat
(7 g trans)
1,950 mg sodium

MENU DECODER

● **CRUMBLIES®:** Fried bits of the batter used to coat the seafood, made mostly of white flour, cornstarch, salt, and spices and served as a side dish.

● **HUSHPUPPIES:** A Southern specialty of deep-fried balls of cornmeal and enriched white flour flavored with dehydrated onion and sugar.

Other Passes

470 calories
23 g fat (8 g saturated)
1,210 mg sodium

Fish Sandwich

270 calories
16 g fat (4 g saturated)
570 mg sodium

Popcorn Shrimp Snack Box

310 calories
22 g fat (13 g saturated)

Chocolate Cream Pie

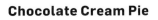

89

Manchu Wok

Did You Know?

● General Tso's Chicken is named after an infamous military leader in China in the 1800s. While no one knows how the general became the namesake of this Westernized Chinese dish, it's a certifiable fact that it's one of the worst items you can order at a Chinese restaurant.

● Noodle dishes are rarely a healthy option—they're made with copious amounts of oil to keep the strands from sticking. Order noodles at Manchu Wok at you'll slurp up 13 grams of fat and 646 mg of sodium.

Eat This

Oriental Grilled Chicken
and Mixed Vegetables

385 calories
18 g fat
(2 g saturated)
1,249 mg sodium

By subbing in vegetables for the standard rice or noodle accompaniment, you cut 180 calories from the meal, plus add a ton of nutrients.

Other Picks

Butterfly Shrimp
and Black Mushroom Tofu

394 calories
17 g fat (2 g saturated)
810 mg sodium

Satay Chicken

211 calories
16 g fat (2 g saturated)
269 mg sodium

Sweet & Sour Pork

271 calories
16 g fat (3 g saturated)
244 mg sodium

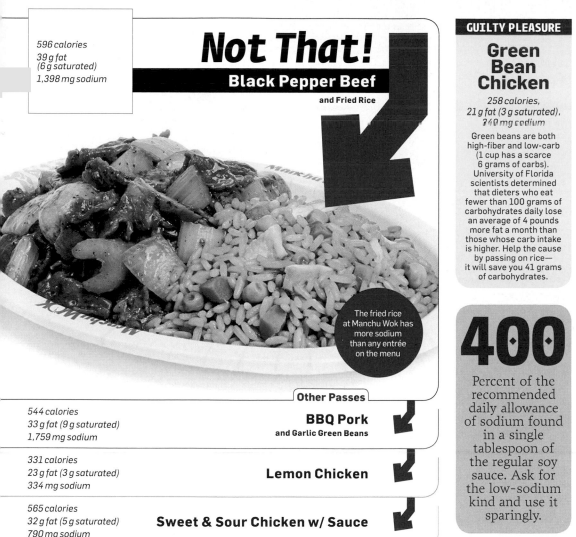

596 calories
39 g fat
(6 g saturated)
1,398 mg sodium

Not That!

Black Pepper Beef

and Fried Rice

The fried rice at Manchu Wok has more sodium than any entrée on the menu

Other Passes

BBQ Pork
and Garlic Green Beans

544 calories
33 g fat (9 g saturated)
1,759 mg sodium

Lemon Chicken

331 calories
23 g fat (3 g saturated)
334 mg sodium

Sweet & Sour Chicken w/ Sauce

565 calories
32 g fat (5 g saturated)
790 mg sodium

GUILTY PLEASURE

Green Bean Chicken

258 calories,
21 g fat (3 g saturated),
?40 mg sodium

Green beans are both high-fiber and low-carb (1 cup has a scarce 6 grams of carbs). University of Florida scientists determined that dieters who eat fewer than 100 grams of carbohydrates daily lose an average of 4 pounds more fat a month than those whose carb intake is higher. Help the cause by passing on rice—it will save you 41 grams of carbohydrates.

400

Percent of the recommended daily allowance of sodium found in a single tablespoon of the regular soy sauce. Ask for the low-sodium kind and use it sparingly.

McDonald's

Did You Know?

● McDonald's is the world's largest purchaser of beef, potatoes, and apples.

● McDonald's opens a new restaurant every four hours.

HIDDEN DANGER

Chicken Selects® Premium Breast Strips (5 pieces) with Creamy Ranch Sauce

The only thing "premium" about these strips is the caloric price you pay. 20 McNuggets® have the same impact. Instead, choose the six-piece offering with BBQ sauce and save yourself 530 calories.

830 calories
55 g fat (4.5 g trans)
48 g carbs

Eat This

Quarter Pounder®

without Cheese

410 calories
19 g fat
(7 g saturated)
730 mg sodium

Sans cheese, the Quarter Pounder® has a good balance of fat, protein, and carbohydrates. Pair it with a side salad and an iced tea and you've got a reasonable meal.

Other Picks

Asian Salad with Grilled Chicken
and Newman's Own® Low-Fat Sesame Dressing

390 calories
12.5 g fat (1 g saturated)
1,630 mg sodium

6 piece Chicken McNuggets®

280 calories
17 g fat (3 g saturated)
600 mg sodium

Egg McMuffin®

300 calories
12 g fat (5 g saturated)
820 mg sodium

Not That!

Premium Grilled Chicken Club
sandwich

570 calories
21 g fat
(7 g saturated)
1,720 mg sodium

Chicken doesn't always trump beef in the health department, especially when it comes robed in bacon, mayo, and liquid margarine.

premium chicken

MENU DECODER

● **BIG MAC® SAUCE:** There's no secret here: this sauce is a mix of soybean oil, pickle relish, vinegar, and egg yolks, along with a dose of high-fructose corn syrup. The sauce adds 190 calories and 9 grams of fat.

● **FILET-O-FISH®:** A battered fish sandwich made of Alaskan pollock, an abundant, mild-flavored member of the cod family found in the Bering Sea. Pollock is the most commonly used fish in breaded and battered retail dishes.

Other Passes

550 calories
32.5 g fat (7.5 g saturated)
1,660 mg sodium

Caesar Salad with Crispy Chicken and Croutons
and Newman's Own® Creamy Caesar Dressing

380 calories
18 g fat (4 g saturated)
640 mg sodium

Filet-O-Fish®

610 calories
18 g fat (4 g saturated)
680 mg sodium

Hotcakes

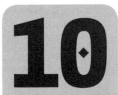

10

Percentage of Americans who have logged time behind the counter at Mickey D's

Olive Garden

Did You Know?

● Since the late 1990s, Olive Garden has pushed a broad wine initiative and now claims to be the leading wine seller among restaurants in the U.S. Managers at each restaurant participate in wine education and training.

GUILTY PLEASURE

Sangria

Vitamin C in the fruit helps bolster your immune system, and resveratrol—the polyphenol found in red wine—can stop influenza cells from replicating, according to scientists at Rome's Institute of Microbiology. Limit yourself to one glass, though, since too much alcohol may impair your immune system.

Eat This

Linguine Alla Marinara

with a Breadstick

691 calories
9.5 g fat
1,040 mg sodium*

*Numbers are approximate; Olive Garden does not provide nutrition information.

Men who ate two to four servings of tomatoes per week reduced their risk of prostate cancer by 26 percent, a study review in the *Journal of Nutrition* found.

Other Picks

Shrimp Primavera

706 calories
18 g fat
1,220 mg sodium

Chicken Giardino

448 calories
11 g fat
1,670 mg sodium

1,315 calories
86 g fat
2,550 mg sodium

Not That!

Stuffed Chicken Marsala

with Garlic Parmesan Mashed Potatoes

This roasted chicken is stuffed with cheese and covered in a Marsala sauce spiked with heavy cream, giving this dish an entire day's worth of fat.

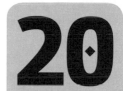

20◆

Percentage fewer calories you'll consume if you start your meal with a soup appetizer, according to a Penn State study.

HIDDEN DANGER

Stuffed Mushrooms

Although mushrooms are normally a healthy side option, this appetizer is stuffed with a deadly trio of cheeses— Parmesan, Romano, and mozzarella— which cancel out any nutritional benefits provided by the fungi.

386 calories
31 g fat
515 mg sodium

Other Passes

839 calories
43 g fat
1,541 mg sodium

Mixed Grill with Vegetables and mashed potatoes

1,011 calories
57 g fat
2,479 mg sodium

Pork Filettino with potatoes and bell peppers

On the Border

Did You Know?

● On the Border's Guacamole Live! and Queso Live! are made to order at your table. Choose the heart-healthy guac over the queso, which consists of meat, creamy cheese sauce, and sour cream.

● Six of the 12 entrées on the Kids Menu contain more than 30 grams of fat.

LITTLE TRICK

Opt for Grilled Vegetables and Black Bean & Corn Relish over the standard rice and refried beans that accompany nearly every meal here and you'll save 390 calories and 1,520 mg of sodium.

Eat This

Chicken Salsa Fresca

510 calories
11g fat
(4 g saturated)
600 mg sodium

> The 49 grams of protein in this dish will work to keep your metabolic fires burning long after the meal.

Other Picks

Jalapeno-BBQ Salmon

530 calories
18 g fat (2.5 g saturated)
1,600 mg sodium

2 Crispy Chicken Tacos
with Grilled Vegetables and Guacamole

590 calories
30 g fat (11 g saturated)
1,630 mg sodium

2 Beef Enchiladas

680 calories
34 g fat (12 g saturated)
1,580 mg sodium

1,150 calories
75 g fat
(24 g saturated)
3,310 mg sodium

Not That!

Blackened Chicken Fiesta Salad

with Chipotle Honey Dressing

The blend of spices used to "blacken" the chicken adds nearly 700 mg of sodium to this dish.

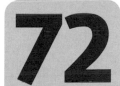

72

Grams of saturated fat found in the Stacked Border Nachos: more than in an entire stick of butter.

WEAPON OF MASS DESTRUCTION

Dos XX® Fish Tacos with Rice and Beans

The Impact:
2,100 calories
130 g fat
(35 g saturated)
4,760 mg sodium

Hands down, the worst fish dish in America. Ask for grilled fish (instead of fried) and replace the rice & beans with veggies, and you'll cut the damage in half.

Other Passes

1,820 calories
107 g fat (38 g saturated)
5,650 mg sodium

Original-Mesquite Grilled Shrimp Fajitas
with Rice, Beans, and all the fixings

1,160 calories
85 g fat (27 g saturated)
2,290 mg sodium

Spicy Chicken Border Chimichanga

1,060 calories
76 g fat (16 g saturated)
1,920 mg sodium

2 Fish Tacos

Outback Steakhouse

Did You Know?

● Founded in Tampa, Outback draws more inspiration from Creoles than Aussies: They rub their steaks with a 17-spice blend and serve their seafood with a Cajun remoulade sauce.

HIDDEN DANGER

Coconut Shrimp

Shrimp is normally a low-fat alternative to loaded burgers and creamy pastas, but the seafood in this dish more closely resembles chicken nuggets. The shrimp is beer battered, rolled in coconut, and then fried.

690 calories
30 g fat

Eat This

Prime Minister's Prime Rib

with Fresh Veggies and Sweet Potato

730 calories
39 g fat
65 g carbohydrates

*Numbers are approximate; Outback Steakhouse does not provide nutrition information.

Sweet potatoes can ward off cancer. Eating two sweet potatoes every week will provide you with beta carotene, which has been shown to decrease skin-cancer risk.

Other Picks

Victoria Filet® (9 oz)
with Steamed Vegetables

639 calories
45 g fat
14 g carbohydrates

Half an Order of Shrimp on the Barbie with Bread

330 calories
21 g fat
32 g carbohydrates

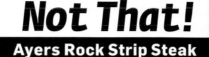

Not That!

Ayers Rock Strip Steak
with Sautéed Mushrooms and Loaded Jacket Potato

1,450 calories
85 g fat
87 g carbohydrates

The stuffed jacket potato alone adds 500 calories to the meal. Go with grilled onions, sauteed mushrooms, or a sweet potato instead.

1665

That's the number of stairs to the top of the Eiffel Tower. You'd have to climb them 2½ times to burn off the 1,150 calories in half a Bloomin' Onion® appetizer.

LITTLE TRICK

You can order any fish or sandwich to be prepared without butter (most are liberally doused in it).

GUILTY PLEASURE

Foster's® Lager

156 calories
11 g carbohydrates

Swedish researchers found that beers with at least 4.5% alcohol (Foster's has 4.9%) can lower your risk of kidney cancer.

Other Passes

Outback Special® (11 oz)
with Sauteed Mushrooms

960 calories
61 g fat
12 g carbohydrates

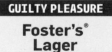

Half a Bloomin' Onion®

1,155 calories
67 g fat
120 g carbohydrates

Panda Express

GUILTY PLEASURE

Chicken Egg Roll

170 calories
8 g fat (1.5 g saturated)

There's not a lot of nutritional benefit to be gained here, but this may be your only chance to eat an egg roll under 300 calories and 10 grams of fat.

Did You Know?

● With more than 800 locations in 35 states, Panda Express is the largest and fastest-growing Chinese restaurant chain in the U.S.

● The only item on Panda Express's menu that contains trans fat is also the most popular, the Orange Chicken. Fortunately, it's but a single gram of this troublesome fat.

Eat This

Broccoli Beef

Mushroom Chicken and Mixed Veggies

350 calories
17 g fat
(3.5 g saturated)
1,200 mg sodium

Opt for broccoli over string beans—broccoli has 6 times more selenium and 5 times more vitamin C than green beans.

Other Picks

Tangy Shrimp

150 calories
5 g fat (1 g saturated)
550 mg sodium

String Bean Chicken Breast

160 calories
8 g fat (1.5 g saturated)
550 mg sodium

Mixed Vegetables

90 calories
7 g fat (1 g saturated)
110 mg sodium

1,060 calories
40.5 g fat
(12.5 g saturated)
2,140 mg sodium

Not That!

Kung Pao Chicken

BBQ Pork and Steamed Rice

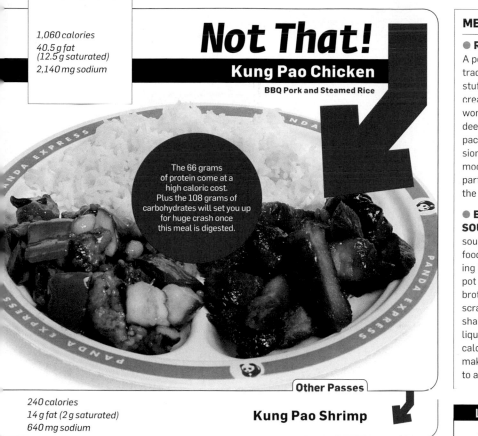

The 66 grams of protein come at a high caloric cost. Plus the 108 grams of carbohydrates will set you up for huge crash once this meal is digested.

MENU DECODER

● **RANGOON:**
A popular appetizer traditionally made by stuffing crab and cream cheese into a won ton wrapper, then deep-frying the whole package. Panda's version drops the only moderately healthy part of the equation—the crab.

● **EGG FLOWER SOUP:** AKA egg drop soup. Chinese comfort food made by streaming beaten eggs into a pot of hot chicken broth so that the eggs scramble in thin shards throughout the liquid. With only 88 calories a serving, it makes a great addition to a meal.

Other Passes

240 calories
14 g fat (2 g saturated)
640 mg sodium

Kung Pao Shrimp

500 calories
27 g fat (5.5 g saturated)
810 mg sodium

Orange Chicken

180 calories
10 g fat (1.5 g saturated)
690 mg sodium

Eggplant and Tofu in Garlic Sauce

LITTLE TRICK

Skip rice and noodles entirely: Even the basic steamed rice has 380 calories and 81 grams of carbohydrates.

Panera

Did You Know?

● Panera bakes more bread each day than any other bakery-cafe in the country.

● Panera operates the country's largest free wireless network, with Wi-Fi offered at most of its locations.

GUILTY PLEASURE

Nutty Oatmeal Raisin Cookie

340 calories
14 g fat (6 g saturated)
21 g sugars

In a smorgasbord of muffins, pastries, and cake, the Nutty Oatmeal Raisin Cookie proves a reasonable indulgence. The oats pack soluble fiber, which helps cut cholesterol, and raisins are rich in potassium, which staves off hypertension. Plus, this cookie has less sugar than any other cookie or muffin.

Eat This
BBQ Chicken Crispani®
(⅓ Pizza)

380 calories
15 g fat (6 g saturated)
980 mg sodium

Crispani®, a line of thin-crust flatbread pizzas, contain fewer calories than any Panera sandwich—between 320 and 380 calories per serving.

Other Picks

Strawberry Poppyseed & Chicken Salad

310 calories
3.5 g fat (0.5 saturated)
530 mg sodium

Low-Fat Vegetarian Garden Vegetable Soup (8 oz)
with a Whole Grain Loaf

220 calories
2.5 g fat (0 g saturated)
1,190 mg sodium

Chai Tea Latte

190 calories
4 g fat (2.5 g saturated)
85 mg sodium

840 calories
40 g fat
(7 g saturated)
2,080 mg sodium

Not That!
Sierra Turkey Sandwich

Love turkey? Try the smoked turkey on sourdough—it has *half* the calories.

How can a turkey sandwich do so much damage? The Asiago Cheese Focaccia bread has 6 grams of fat per slice, and the turkey's slathered in chipotle mayo.

WEAPON OF MASS DESTRUCTION

Italian Combo Sandwich

The Impact:
1,100 calories
56 g fat (20 g saturated)
3,200 mg sodium

The bread alone yields 82 carbs. Instead, choose one kind of meat, and substitute a whole grain baguette or loaf.

MENU DECODER

● **MUFFIE:** The top half of a muffin, in flavors like chocolate chip and pumpkin, for half the saturated fat of the whole muffin.

LITTLE TRICK

Order your soup with a sourdough roll instead of a gargantuan bread bowl—you'll cut 370 calories from your meal.

Other Passes

580 calories
30 g fat (7 g saturated)
1,020 mg sodium

Fuji Apple Chicken Salad

790 calories
17.5 g fat (9 g saturated)
2,210 mg sodium

Broccoli Cheddar Soup (8 oz)
in a Sourdough Soup Bowl

390 calories
16 g fat (10 g saturated)
200 mg sodium

Caramel Latte

Papa John's

Did You Know?

● Papa John's was one of the first major pizza chains to include a dipping sauce with each delivery. The eight flavors, like Blue Cheese and Special Garlic, can carry up to 18 grams of fat, so choose wisely—the Pizza and Barbeque dipping sauces do the least damage.

LITTLE TRICK

Add kick to your pizza with a packet of crushed red pepper. It's fat free, and the capsaicin in the pepper has been shown to stimulate metabolism.

Eat This

Two Slices Original Crust Spinach Alfredo Pizza (12")

400 calories
16 g fat
(6 g saturated)
900 mg sodium

Spinach contains vitamins A, C, K, and folate, and minerals like calcium and magnesium to ward off cancer, heart disease, and stroke.

Other Picks

Two slices Thin Crust Cheese Pizza (14")

480 calories
26 g fat (7 g saturated)
1,000 mg sodium

Two slices Original Crust Garden Fresh Pizza (12")

400 calories
14 g fat (4 g saturated)
980 mg sodium

Breadsticks (2)
with Pizza dipping sauce

300 calories
4 g fat (0 g saturated)
660 mg sodium

760 calories
30 g fat
(14 g saturated)
1,960 mg sodium

Not That!

Two Slices Pan Crust Cheese Pizza (12")

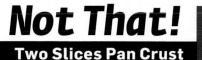

NEW!

Thick Golden Crust
Crispy on the o...
chewy on the...

PAPA

Pan crust has 12 more grams of carbs and 4.5 more grams of saturated fat per slice than Original.

...redients. Better Pizza...
..., A Better Pan!

#1
In Customer Satisfaction
7 Years Straight!

Other Passes

700 calories
32 g fat (10 g saturated)
1,840 mg sodium

Two slices Original Crust The Meats Pizza (14")

520 calories
16 g fat (14 g saturated)
1,360 mg sodium

Two slices Original Crust Spicy Italian Pizza (12")

520 calories
33 g fat (7.5 g saturated)
1,140 mg sodium

Cheesesticks (2)
with Special Garlic dipping sauce

MENU DECODER

● **GARDEN FRESH:** Papa John's doesn't used vacuum-packed, pre-cut vegetables on their pizzas. The Garden Fresh pizza is topped with mushrooms, black olives from southern Spain, green peppers, onions, and roma tomatoes. The green peppers and onions are purchased in local markets and sliced fresh at the restaurants.

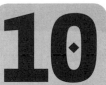

10

Number of miles you'd have to cross-country ski to burn the 1,570 calories in a Papa John's Hawaiian BBQ Chicken pizza with a 20-ounce Coke®. It would take you 1 hour and 49 minutes.

Pizza Hut

Did You Know?

● A standard pizza in Italy contains 500 to 800 calories. A medium cheese pizza at Pizza Hut has up to 2,160 calories. Approximate Italy by ordering your next pie with a thin crust, half the cheese, and extra vegetables.

HIDDEN DANGER

Wing Dipping Sauce

Both the blue cheese and the ranch sauces have twice the calories and 16 more grams of fat than a serving of the wings themselves.

220 calories
23 g fat (4 g saturated)
400 mg sodium

Eat This

Two Slices Thin 'N Crispy Pizza
with Quartered Ham & Pineapple (12")

360 calories
12 g fat
(6 g saturated)
1,140 mg sodium

Pineapple is loaded with bromelain and papain, enzymes that help break down proteins for digestion and have anti-inflammatory properties to help you recover faster from a workout.

Other Picks

Two slices Fit n' Delicious™
Green Pepper, Red Onion & Diced Tomato Pizza (12")

300 calories
8 g fat (3 g saturated)
840 mg sodium

Two slices Thin 'N Crispy
Pepperoni & Mushroom Pizza (12")

380 calories
16 g fat (7 g saturated)
1,120 mg sodium

Cinnamon Sticks (2 pieces)
with White Icing Dipping Cup

320 calories
5 g fat (1 g saturated)
180 mg sodium

620 calories
32 g fat
(12 g saturated)
1,440 mg sodium

Not That!

Two Slices Supreme Pan Pizza (12")

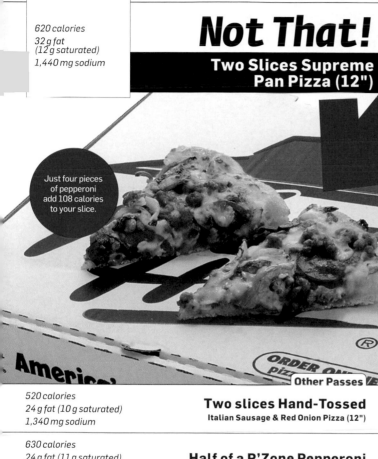

Just four pieces of pepperoni add 108 calories to your slice.

America'

ORDER ONLINE
pizza ®

Other Passes

520 calories
24 g fat (10 g saturated)
1,340 mg sodium

Two slices Hand-Tossed
Italian Sausage & Red Onion Pizza (12")

630 calories
24 g fat (11 g saturated)
1,490 mg sodium

Half of a P'ZONE Pepperoni

340 calories
30 g fat (6 g saturated)
900 mg sodium

Hot Wings (2 pieces)
with Wing Ranch dipping sauce

LITTLE TRICK

Trick yourself into portion control: Cut oversized slices of pizza in half, and eat off a small plate instead of straight from the extra-large-sized box. Studies show that the larger the container, the smaller we invariably consider the portion contained within, which leads to overeating.

MENU DECODER

● **P'ZONE:** Weighing in at over a pound, the P'Zone seals meat toppings and cheese inside a folded-over 12-inch pizza crust.

● **QUEPAPAS® POTATO BITES:** Deadly potato bites filled with cheese and jalapeño, deep-fried and served with fatty ranch dipping sauce.

P. F. Chang's

Did You Know?

● P. F. Chang's states that their goal is to help diners attain a balance of two Chinese food principles: *fan*, which includes starches like rice, noodles, and dumplings, and *t'sai*, meaning vegetables, meat, and seafood. Want to eat better? Disrupt the balance and stick with *t'sai*.

LITTLE TRICK

Have them serve your stir-fry dishes over shredded lettuce instead of noodles or rice—you'll save up to 400 calories and a boatload of carbs in a single meal.

Eat This

Wild Alaskan Sockeye

Steamed with Ginger

750 calories
50 g fat
(8 g saturated)
23 g carbohydrates

Most of the fat in this dish comes from omega-3 fatty acids, a heart-healthy fat commonly found in salmon and other types of fish. The 59 grams of protein will help keep you feeling full long after the plate has passed.

Other Picks

Seared Ahi Tuna

260 calories
6 g fat (0.5 g saturated)
21 g carbohydrates

Ginger Chicken & Broccoli

660 calories
26 g fat (3.5 g saturated)
45 g carbohydrates

Sichuan-Style Asparagus

200 calories
6 g fat (0.5 g saturated)
34 g carbohydrates

1,130 calories
46 g fat
(7 g saturated)
163 g carbohydrates

Not That!
Sriracha Shrimp Salad

WEAPON OF MASS DESTRUCTION

Lo Mein Pork

The Impact:
1,820 calories
127 g fat
(23 g saturated fat)

A wok full of oil sinks this dish. Try the Singapore Street Noodles: The 570 calories and 16 grams of fat stack up well next to this atrocity.

Candied papaya and a sugar-laden dressing push the carb count into the stratosphere.

MENU DECODER

● **SRIRACHA:** This spicy red chile paste is used as a table condiment and to flavor sauces and stir fries across Asia.

Other Passes

770 calories
50 g fat (4 g saturated)
28 g carbohydrates

Salt & Pepper Calamari

1,240 calories
80 g fat (10 g saturated)
58 g carbohydrates

Kung Pao Chicken

610 calories
40 g fat (6 g saturated)
48 g carbohydrates

Spicy Green Beans

GUILTY PLEASURE

Almond Cashew Chicken

740 calories
23 g fat (3.5 g saturated)

Almonds and cashews are both good sources of antioxidants and are high in heart-healthy monounsaturated fats.

Popeyes

Did You Know?

● Started in Louisiana in 1972, Popeyes menu is heavily tinged with the chile-inflected cuisine of the Deep South, so expect a kick in most of the dishes served here.

● The restaurant isn't named after the sailor, but for Popeye Doyle, the drunk cop in "The French Connection."

LITTLE TRICK

Replace the biscuit included in the chicken meals with a third side, like green beans. The biscuit alone has 240 calories and 13 grams of fat.

Eat This

Spicy Chicken Breast

Thigh, Leg, and Wing, Skinless and Breading Removed

290 calories
8.5 g fat
(3 g saturated)
810 mg sodium

Nix the skin and you can eat half a chicken and still take in nearly a third of the fat of a single breaded breast.

Other Picks

2 Mild Chicken Strips

250 calories
10 g fat (4.5 g saturated)
1,080 mg sodium

Crawfish Etouffee (side)

180 calories
5 g fat (1 g saturated)
640 mg sodium

Mashed Potatoes & Gravy

120 calories
4 g fat (2 g saturated)
570 mg sodium

360 calories
22 g fat
(8 g saturated)
760 mg sodium

Not That!
Spicy Chicken Breast

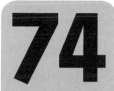

74

Percentage of your recommended daily intake (RDI) of fat found in just six chicken wings at Popeyes.

Popeyes Spicy Chicken Breast has 2 more grams of fat than the mild chicken breast, but 370 mg less sodium.

MENU DECODER

● **JAMBALAYA:** The Cajun version of paella, jambalaya combines chicken, smoked sausage, rice, and a blend of piquant spices. Popeyes uses chicken sausage in their rendition, which keeps the fat to a reasonable 11 grams per serving in a side portion.

● **ETOUFFEE:** A spicy Creole stew made with crawfish, cayenne pepper, and thickened with roux, a mixture of flour and oil.

Other Passes

390 calories
27 g fat (9.5 g saturated)
990 mg sodium

Mild Thigh & Leg

220 calories
11 g fat (3 g saturated)
760 mg sodium

Chicken & Sausage Jambalaya (side)

310 calories
17 g fat (7 g saturated)
660 mg sodium

French Fries

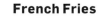

111

Quiznos

Did You Know?

● Quiznos is the second-largest sandwich chain in America, behind Subway. They are the last major sub franchise to offer nutritional information for their sandwiches.

HIDDEN DANGER

Classic Cobb Flatbread Salad

It sounds like a healthy choice, but bacon, bleu cheese crumbles, and ranch dressing tips the scale on this salad. Order yours without the wall of flatbread to cut back on calories and carbs.

960 calories
62 g fat
2,070 mg sodium

Eat This

Small Honey Bourbon Chicken on Wheat Bread

310 calories
4 g fat
(1 g saturated)
920 mg sodium

Opt for the honey bourbon mustard sauce over mayo or creamy dressings to add flavor without guilt.

Other Picks

Small Black Angus Sandwich

520 calories
16.5 g fat (7 g saturated)
1,550 mg sodium

Small Tuscan Turkey
on Rosemary Parmesan without cheese

390 calories
14 g fat (3 g saturated)
1,185 mg sodium

550 calories
30 g fat
(5.5 g saturated)
1,140 mg sodium

Not That!

Small Honey Mustard Chicken Sub

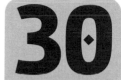

30

The distance, in miles, across the state of Delaware. You'd have to bicycle it to burn 1,510 calories in a large Chicken Carbonara.

GUILTY PLEASURE

Small Traditional Sandwich

430 calories
21 g fat

Even with three kinds of meat, cheese, and ranch dressing, this is still one of the healthiest items on the menu.

One word can change everything. Here, it means bacon and Swiss, which account for the 200-calorie gap between these two sandwiches.

LITTLE TRICK

Make Jimmy's Batch 81 Three Pepper Chili Sauce your best friend. Use it as a spread instead of the ranch or Italian and save a few hundred calories.

Other Passes

680 calories
42 g fat (9 g saturated)
1,070 mg sodium

Small Prime Rib Cheesesteak

450 calories
22.5 g fat (3.5 g saturated)
1,380 mg sodium

Small Turkey Ranch & Swiss Sandwich

Red Lobster

Did You Know?

● Red Lobster does not serve over-fished species like Chilean sea bass, and it participates in conservation efforts such as placing a moratorium on the purchase of grouper during late February and early March. The chain never sells live lobsters that are larger than 4 pounds.

LITTLE TRICK

Request your baked potato with a scoop of pico de gallo instead of butter and sour cream. Besides saving you a few hundred calories, the tomato salsa also provides a dose of powerful antioxidants.

Eat This

Live Maine Lobster (1.25 lbs)

with Cocktail Sauce and Seasoned Broccoli

288 calories
3 g fat
29 g carbs*

*Numbers are approximate; Red Lobster does not provide nutrition information.

Lobsters are a good source of phosphorus, which helps the body to turn carbs and fat into energy and use protein to repair cells and tissues.

Other Picks

Garlic Grilled Jumbo Shrimp
with lemon juice and a baked potato with pico de gallo

329 calories
5 g fat
39 g carbohydrates

Broiled Flounder
with lemon juice and a Garden Salad with red wine vinaigrette

344 calories
10 g fat
15 g carbohydrates

883 calories
35 g fat
36 g carbs

Not That!

North Pacific King Crab Legs

with melted butter and Wild Rice Pilaf

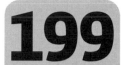

Crab is naturally low in fat and calories, but introduce a coat of butter to each bite and this otherwise healthy meal takes a turn for the worse.

199

Number of minutes you'd have to spend raking the lawn to burn the 1,060 calories in an Admiral's Feast of fried shrimp, scallops, clam strips, and flounder.

HIDDEN DANGER

Melted Butter

Seafood is a great source of heart healthy omega-3s, but not when it's drenched in butter. One fluid ounce drizzles on another 21 grams of fat. Ask for a lemon wedge or cocktail sauce instead to flavor your fish.

Other Passes

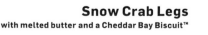

611 calories
34.5 g fat
17 g carbohydrates

Snow Crab Legs

with melted butter and a Cheddar Bay Biscuit™

1,170 calories
66 g fat
1,070 mg sodium

Crab Alfredo

115

Romano's Macaroni Grill

Did You Know?

● Not a single pasta selection on Macaroni Grill's menu has less than 50 grams of fat or 1,200 milligrams of sodium. Cut down on both, and shed 200 calories, by ordering lunch pasta portions at dinner.

4992

Possible pasta combinations with Macaroni Grill's Create Your Own Pasta option. Our favorite: Whole wheat penne with grilled chicken, broccoli, mushrooms, and spicy arrabbiata sauce.

Eat This

½ Pizza Margherita

and Caesar Della Casa with Low-Fat Caesar Dressing

645 calories
24 g fat
(11 g saturated)
1,665 mg sodium

Split a whole pizza with a dining partner and pair it with a salad for an entrée and you'll save yourself some serious calories.

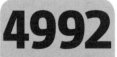

Other Picks

Pollo Magro

330 calories
5 g fat (1 g saturated)
770 mg sodium

Simple Salmon

590 calories
40 g fat (6 g saturated)
1,390 mg sodium

Half Order of Mozzarella Alla Caprese

260 calories
21 g fat (7 g saturated)
410 mg sodium

Not That!

Chicken Caesar

920 calories
69 g fat
(16 g saturated)
1,660 mg sodium

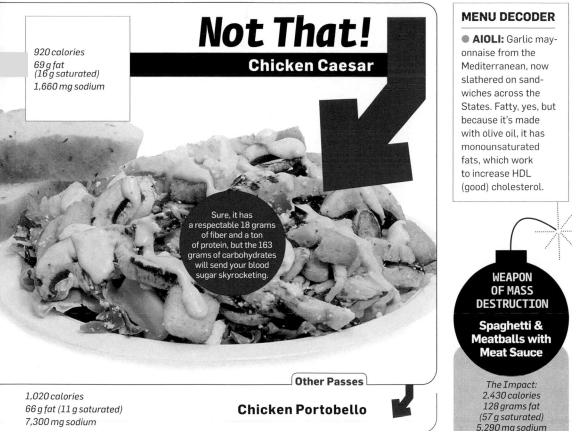

Sure, it has a respectable 18 grams of fiber and a ton of protein, but the 163 grams of carbohydrates will send your blood sugar skyrocketing.

Other Passes

1,020 calories
66 g fat (11 g saturated)
7,300 mg sodium

Chicken Portobello

1,230 calories
74 g fat (9 g saturated)
6,590 mg sodium

Grilled Salmon Teriyaki

440 calories
31.5 g fat (9 g saturated)
885 mg sodium

Half Order of Mozzarella Fritta

MENU DECODER

● **AIOLI:** Garlic mayonnaise from the Mediterranean, now slathered on sandwiches across the States. Fatty, yes, but because it's made with olive oil, it has monounsaturated fats, which work to increase HDL (good) cholesterol.

WEAPON OF MASS DESTRUCTION

Spaghetti & Meatballs with Meat Sauce

The Impact:
2,430 calories
128 grams fat
(57 g saturated)
5,290 mg sodium

With three times your recommended daily intake of saturated fat and two days' worth of salt, these ain't your mama's meatballs (at least we hope not).

Ruby Tuesday

Did You Know?

● Ruby Tuesday prides itself on the quality of its "handcrafted" burgers, which is really just a fancy way of saying someone slaps the beef into a patty before tossing it on the grill. Delicious or not, not a single burger on the menu has fewer than 750 calories or 45 grams of fat.

LITTLE TRICK

Try Creamy Mashed Cauliflower as an alternative to the Mashed Potatoes: You'll get the same rich, smooth texture with 120 fewer calories, half the carbohydrates, and an extra shot of fiber.

Eat This

7 oz Top Sirloin

with Premium Baby Green Beans
and Sautéed Baby Portabella Mushrooms

464 calories
24 g fat*

*Ruby Tuesday does not disclose saturated fat or sodium content.

The Steamed Broccoli that normally comes with this dish has more fat than the steak. Cut 330 calories from the meal by replacing it and the baked potato with green beans and bellas.

Other Picks

Creole Catch with Couscous
and Premium Baby Green Beans

580 calories
26 g fat

Asian Dumplings
(4 dumplings)

440 calories
20 g fat

White Bean Chicken Chili
and Tomato and Mozzarella Salad

370 calories
15 g fat

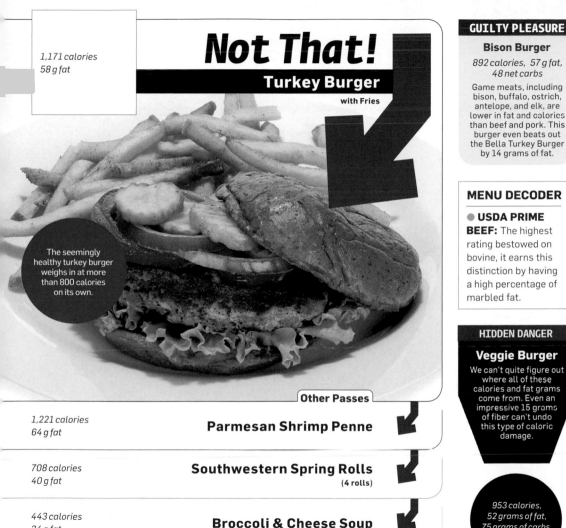

1,171 calories
58 g fat

Not That!
Turkey Burger
with Fries

The seemingly healthy turkey burger weighs in at more than 800 calories on its own.

Other Passes

1,221 calories
64 g fat

Parmesan Shrimp Penne

708 calories
40 g fat

Southwestern Spring Rolls
(4 rolls)

443 calories
34 g fat

Broccoli & Cheese Soup

GUILTY PLEASURE

Bison Burger

892 calories, 57 g fat, 48 net carbs

Game meats, including bison, buffalo, ostrich, antelope, and elk, are lower in fat and calories than beef and pork. This burger even beats out the Bella Turkey Burger by 14 grams of fat.

MENU DECODER

● **USDA PRIME BEEF:** The highest rating bestowed on bovine, it earns this distinction by having a high percentage of marbled fat.

HIDDEN DANGER

Veggie Burger

We can't quite figure out where all of these calories and fat grams come from. Even an impressive 15 grams of fiber can't undo this type of caloric damage.

953 calories, 52 grams of fat, 75 grams of carbs.

119

Sbarro

Did You Know?

● Sbarro began as an Italian grocery store in Brooklyn, selling mozzarella, imported cheese, sausage, and salami. It now has nearly 1,000 outlets in 30 countries.

HIDDEN DANGER

Stuffed Eggplant

Eggplant is high in vitamins and minerals and protects your brain against free radical damage. Here, however, the purple veggie is "overstuffed" with ricotta, mozzarella, and Romano cheeses and served on a bed of spaghetti with a breadstick.

Eat This

One slice Low Carb Cheese Pizza

with a Fruit Salad (12 oz)

440 calories
15 g fat
655 mg sodium*

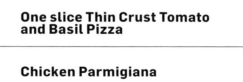

*Numbers are approximate; Sbarro does not provide nutrition information.

Watermelon increases levels of arginine, an amino acid that boosts bloodflow to your heart.

Other Picks

One slice Thin Crust Tomato and Basil Pizza

450 calories
14 g fat
1,040 mg sodium

Chicken Parmigiana

520 calories
22 g fat
750 mg sodium

One slice Thin Crust Chicken and Vegetable Pizza

530 calories
17 g fat
1,260 mg sodium

790 calories
32 g fat
1,545 mg sodium

Not That!

One slice Deep Dish Cheese Pizza

with a Cucumber and Tomato Salad (8 oz)

Sbarro's deep dish is topped with a combination of mozzarella and Romano cheese, upping the fat and sodium content. This particular combo also has 93 grams of carbohydrates.

WEAPON OF MASS DESTRUCTION

Pepperoni Stromboli

The Impact:
890 calories
44 g fat
2,470 mg sodium

This mozzarella- and pepperoni-packed pocket of dough delivers more than 100 percent of your daily sodium allowance.

MENU DECODER

● **PIZZA BLANCA:** Pizza topped with ricotta cheese instead of tomato sauce, which adds 10 grams of fat to a slice.

LITTLE TRICK

Lasagna clocks 650 calories and 37 g of fat. Add an onion-rich salad to cut cholesterol after the double onslaught of cheese and meat.

Other Passes

730 calories
37 g fat
2,200 mg sodium

One slice Thin Crust Pepperoni Pizza

650 calories
37 g fat
1,130 mg sodium

Meat Lasagna

770 calories
28 g fat
1,410 mg sodium

Cheese Calzone

121

Schlotzsky's

Did You Know?

● Schlotzsky's began in 1971 as a mom-and-pop shop serving only a single sandwich, The Original®, which is still their most popular sandwich today. Made with ham, two types of salami, and three cheeses, it's also one of the least healthy items on the menu.

GUILTY PLEASURE

Grilled Chicken and Guacamole Wrap

667 calories
36 g fat
1,391 mg sodium

Most of the fat and calories come from the avocado in the guacamole. Fortunately, the avocado fat is monounsaturated, the good-for-your-heart-kind that helps lower LDL (bad) cholesterol.

Eat This

Mediterranean Tuna Wrap

440 calories
14 g fat
1,304 mg sodium*

*Schlotzsky's does not provide saturated fat data.

The tuna is bound in a fat-free spicy ranch dressing, making this a healthier option than traditional tuna salad.

Other Picks

Small Smoked Turkey Breast Sandwich	*345 calories* *5 g fat* *1,240 mg sodium*
Fresh Tomato & Pesto Pizza	*556 calories* *19 g fat* *1,334 mg sodium*
Cup of Hearty Vegetable Beef Soup and Side Salad	*135 calories* *6 g fat* *1,256 mg sodium*

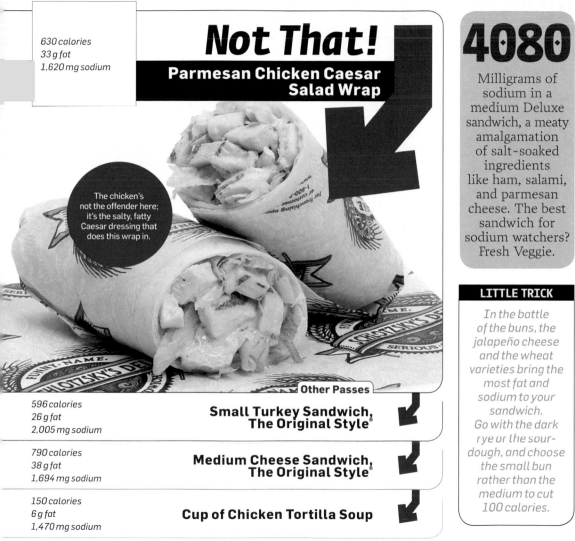

630 calories
33 g fat
1,620 mg sodium

Not That!
Parmesan Chicken Caesar Salad Wrap

The chicken's not the offender here; it's the salty, fatty Caesar dressing that does this wrap in.

4080

Milligrams of sodium in a medium Deluxe sandwich, a meaty amalgamation of salt-soaked ingredients like ham, salami, and parmesan cheese. The best sandwich for sodium watchers? Fresh Veggie.

LITTLE TRICK

In the battle of the buns, the jalapeño cheese and the wheat varieties bring the most fat and sodium to your sandwich. Go with the dark rye or the sourdough, and choose the small bun rather than the medium to cut 100 calories.

Other Passes

596 calories
26 g fat
2,005 mg sodium

Small Turkey Sandwich, The Original Style®

790 calories
38 g fat
1,694 mg sodium

Medium Cheese Sandwich, The Original Style®

150 calories
6 g fat
1,470 mg sodium

Cup of Chicken Tortilla Soup

123

Smoothie King

Did You Know?

● Most of Smoothie King's offerings are sweetened with honey and turbinado, unprocessed cane sugar more commonly known as Sugar in the Raw. While these may offer some flavor benefits, both sweeteners have a similarly adverse impact on your insulin levels (and your waistline) as regular sugar.

LITTLE TRICK

Order your smoothie "skinny" to leave out the turbinado, saving you 100 calories and 23 grams of carbs.

Eat This

Amaretto Coffee Smoothie
(20 oz)

118 calories
0 g fat
13 g sugars

Coffee is the number-one source of antioxidants in the American diet.

SMOOTHIE KING

Other Picks

Pineapple Pleasure Smoothie
(20 oz)

313 calories
0.5 g fat (0 g saturated)
52 g sugars

Slim-N-Trim Vanilla Smoothie
(20 oz)

227 calories
1 g fat (.5 g saturated)
44 g sugars

Celestial Cherry High Smoothie
(20 oz)

285 calories
0.5 g fat (0 g saturated)
36 g sugars

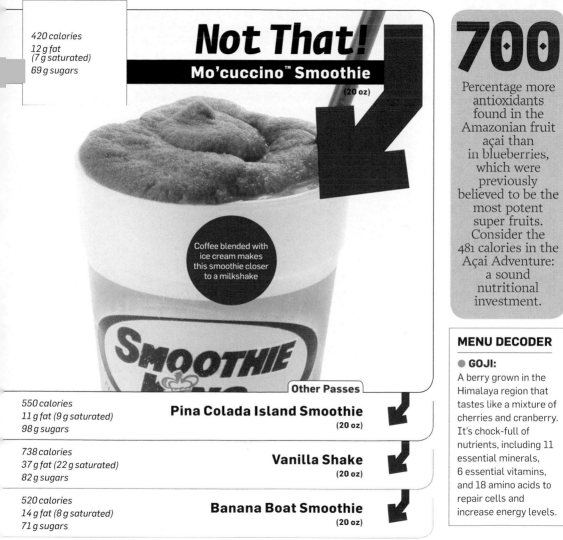

420 calories
12 g fat
(7 g saturated)
69 g sugars

Not That!

Mo'cuccino™ Smoothie

(20 oz)

Coffee blended with ice cream makes this smoothie closer to a milkshake

700

Percentage more antioxidants found in the Amazonian fruit açai than in blueberries, which were previously believed to be the most potent super fruits. Consider the 481 calories in the Açai Adventure: a sound nutritional investment.

MENU DECODER

● **GOJI:**
A berry grown in the Himalaya region that tastes like a mixture of cherries and cranberry. It's chock-full of nutrients, including 11 essential minerals, 6 essential vitamins, and 18 amino acids to repair cells and increase energy levels.

Other Passes

550 calories
11 g fat (9 g saturated)
98 g sugars

Pina Colada Island Smoothie
(20 oz)

738 calories
37 g fat (22 g saturated)
82 g sugars

Vanilla Shake
(20 oz)

520 calories
14 g fat (8 g saturated)
71 g sugars

Banana Boat Smoothie
(20 oz)

Sonic

Did You Know?

● The name Sonic came from the restaurant's original slogan, "service at the speed of sound," a reference to the speaker boxes used in the original drive-ins. Sonic still uses a PA system for ordering and carhops (sometimes on roller skates) to deliver the food.

LITTLE TRICK

Try the Grilled Chicken Sandwich with marinara instead of mayo. It has twice the flavor, a dose of cancer-fighting lycopene, and will save you 9 grams of fat.

Eat This

Sonic® Burger with Mustard

540 calories
25 g fat
(9 g saturated)
730 mg sodium

Cut 25 percent of the fat by picking mustard over mayo.

Other Picks

Grilled Chicken on Ciabatta
with BBQ sauce

375 calories
9 g fat (1.5 g saturated)
1,310 mg sodium

Grilled Chicken Wrap

380 calories
11 g fat (2.5 g saturated)
1,300 mg sodium

Junior Banana Split

200 calories
4.5 g fat (3.5 g saturated)
27 g sugars

690 calories
35 g fat
(10 g saturated)
1,900 mg sodium

Not That!

Chicken Club
Toaster® Sandwich

HIDDEN DANGER

**Minute Maid®
Cranberry
Juice Slush**

Cranberry juice is the
Ryan Seacrest of
drinks—fine in small
doses, but too sickly
sweet to pour on
heavy. A large has
more sugar than
3 sodas.

450 calories
124 g sugars

How can a chicken
sandwich pack so much fat?
Start with a fried chicken
breast, add bacon,
cheese, and mayo, and
you're there. Ditch the swine
and save 10 grams
of fat.

Other Passes

490 calories
28 g fat (9 g saturated)
1,440 mg sodium

Jumbo Popcorn Chicken® Salad

640 calories
31 g fat (5 g saturated)
1,180 mg sodium

Fish Sandwich

290 calories
0 g fat
77 g sugars

Large Hi-C® Fruit Punch

MENU DECODER

● **ONION RINGS:**
Nothing irregular
here—onions, batter,
hot fat—except
these crispy Os might
be the only ones
left in the fast food
world that are still
made fresh by hand.
Delicious? Maybe.
But a large order
packs a punishing
720 calories and 41
grams of fat.

127

Starbucks

Did You Know?

● Starbucks is adopting new dairy standards for all espresso-based drinks, switching from whole milk to 2% in all Starbucks stores in the U.S. and Canada by the end of 2007.

WEAPON OF MASS DESTRUCTION

Venti® White Hot Chocolate
with whipped cream (whole milk)

The Impact:
640 calories
28 g fat (18 g saturated)
76 g sugars

A meal in a cup. Cut fat by asking for skim milk and slash added sugars by requesting one pump of syrup instead of the usual three or four.

Eat This

Black Forest Ham, Egg, and Cheddar Breakfast Sandwich

with a Grande Sugar-Free Nonfat Vanilla Lattè

510 calories
16 g fat (8 g saturated)
21 g sugars

Ordering your lattè with sugar-free syrup and without whip knocks 37 grams of sugar off your drink and staves off a mid-morning crash.

Careful, the beverage you're about to enjoy is extremely hot.

Other Picks

French Toast Bagel

280 calories
1 g fat (0 g saturated)
10 g sugars

Grande Dulce de Leche Frappuccino® Light

170 calories
0.5 g fat (0 g saturated)
25 g sugars

Grande Nonfat Caffè Latte
with a shot of Caramel Syrup

150 calories
0 g fat (0 g saturated)
23 g sugars

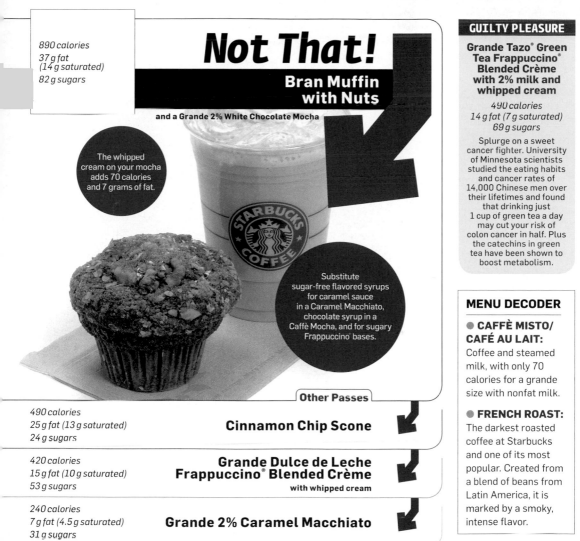

890 calories
37 g fat
(14 g saturated)
82 g sugars

Not That!

Bran Muffin with Nuts

and a Grande 2% White Chocolate Mocha

The whipped cream on your mocha adds 70 calories and 7 grams of fat.

Substitute sugar-free flavored syrups for caramel sauce in a Caramel Macchiato, chocolate syrup in a Caffè Mocha, and for sugary Frappuccino bases.

Other Passes

490 calories
25 g fat (13 g saturated)
24 g sugars

Cinnamon Chip Scone

420 calories
15 g fat (10 g saturated)
53 g sugars

Grande Dulce de Leche Frappuccino® Blended Crème
with whipped cream

240 calories
7 g fat (4.5 g saturated)
31 g sugars

Grande 2% Caramel Macchiato

GUILTY PLEASURE

Grande Tazo® Green Tea Frappuccino® Blended Crème with 2% milk and whipped cream

490 calories
14 g fat (7 g saturated)
69 g sugars

Splurge on a sweet cancer fighter. University of Minnesota scientists studied the eating habits and cancer rates of 14,000 Chinese men over their lifetimes and found that drinking just 1 cup of green tea a day may cut your risk of colon cancer in half. Plus the catechins in green tea have been shown to boost metabolism.

MENU DECODER

● **CAFFÈ MISTO/ CAFÉ AU LAIT:**
Coffee and steamed milk, with only 70 calories for a grande size with nonfat milk.

● **FRENCH ROAST:**
The darkest roasted coffee at Starbucks and one of its most popular. Created from a blend of beans from Latin America, it is marked by a smoky, intense flavor.

Subway

Did You Know?

● Any sandwich on the Subway menu can be prepared as a salad.

● A recent study found that subjects ate 350 calories more at Subway than they did at McDonald's. Researchers call it the "health halo": the tendency for diners to overeat when they believe they're eating at a healthy restaurant.

LITTLE TRICK

Looking to cut down on the salt? Stick with Swiss cheese. It has one-third the sodium of cheddar, and one-fourth the sodium of provolone.

Eat This

6-inch Double Roast Beef Sub

360 calories
7 g fat
(3.5 g saturated)
1,300 mg sodium

Want an exciting stand-in for mayo? Try the Sweet Onion Sauce or the Honey Mustard. Both go well with nearly everything and will spare you 12 grams of fat.

Even with twice the meat—and double the protein—this sandwich still has only a fraction of the fat found in the tuna.

Other Picks

6-inch Steak & Cheese

400 calories
12 g fat (6 g saturated)
1,110 mg sodium

Oven Roasted Chicken Breast Salad
with Fat Free Italian Dressing

175 calories
2.5 g fat (0.5 g saturated)
1,120 mg sodium

Roasted Chicken Noodle Soup

80 calories
2 g fat (0.5 g saturated)
1,240 mg sodium

530 calories
31 g fat
(7 g saturated)
1,010 mg sodium

Not That!
6-inch Tuna Sub

Gloppy mayo-based tuna salad sends this sandwich's fat counts skyrocketing.

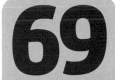

69

Cost, in cents, of a sub at the founding Subway location in 1965.

GUILTY PLEASURE

Chili Con Carne

*290 calories
8 g fat (3.5 g saturated)
990 mg sodium*

The beans contain selenium and 12 grams of fiber, while the beef gives you a protein boost with 19 grams. And Tulane University researchers found that eating beans four times a week can lower the risk of heart disease by 19 percent.

LITTLE TRICK

Rather than order a large sub, double up on your meat on a small. You'll save more than cash: Try this with a turkey sandwich and save 230 calories.

Other Passes

560 calories
24 g fat (11 g saturated)
1,590 mg sodium

Meatball Marinara

430 calories
37.5 g fat (6.5 g saturated)
1,140 mg sodium

Turkey Breast Salad
with Ranch Dressing

210 calories
11 g fat (4 g saturated)
1,250 mg sodium

Wild Rice with Chicken Soup

131

Taco Bell

Did You Know?

● Taco Bell switched over to trans fat-free frying oil in April of 2007. Still, watch out for the nachos and the taco salads; both of these entrées still contain an unhealthy dose of this heart-threatening fat.

GUILTY PLEASURE

Bean Burrito

340 calories
9 g fat (3.5 g saturated)
1,190 mg sodium

Arizona State University researchers found that $1/2$ cup of pinto beans daily can cut LDL (bad) cholesterol by 8 percent, which happens to be the same amount found in a bean burrito. Ask for it "fresco" style and slice off extra calories and sodium.

Eat This

Two Grilled Steak Soft Tacos, Fresco Style

320 calories
9 g fat
(3 g saturated)
1,100 mg sodium

Order almost any menu item "fresco" style and the Bell boys will replace cheese and sauces with a chunky tomato salsa, helping to cut calories dramatically and fat by at least 25 percent.

Other Picks

Chicken Fiesta Taco Salad
without shell

470 calories
24 g fat (10 g saturated)
1,780 mg sodium

Two Spicy Chicken Soft Tacos

340 calories
12 g fat (4 g saturated)
1,160 mg sodium

Cinnamon Twists

170 calories
7 g fat (0 g saturated)
200 mg sodium

410 calories
27 g fat
(6 g saturated)
780 mg sodium

Not That!

Baja Beef Chalupa

370

Number of calories you'll save by ditching the oversized shell with your next taco salad. You'll also cut 20 grams of fat.

The Chalupa shell alone has 13 grams of fat and 25 grams of carbs.

MENU DECODER

● **BAJA SAUCE:**
A spicy, mayo-based sauce loaded with saturated fat, which makes it the worst choice for a gordita or chalupa. The lesser of the evils, surprisingly, is the nacho cheese.

● **CHALUPA:**
In Taco Bell parlance, a chalupa is deep-fried flatbread fashioned into a taco shell to hold meat, sauce, cheese, and some token produce. Chalupas have 70 calories and 7 grams more fat than gorditas.

Other Passes

640 calories
35 g fat (6 g saturated)
1,800 mg sodium

Zesty Chicken BORDER BOWL®

640 calories
23 g fat (7 g saturated)
2,160 mg sodium

Grilled Stuft Chicken Burrito

290 calories
14 g fat (2.5 g saturated)
300 mg sodium

Caramel Apple Empanadas

133

Uno Chicago Grill

Did You Know?

● In 1998, Uno's unleashed the Bigger and Better menu, featuring new entrées and larger portions. Today, if you cut an individual serving of Uno's Chicago Classic Deep Dish in half, you would still be consuming more than 100 percent of your daily allotment of fat.

LITTLE TRICK

Hunt for the word "grilled" on the menu: the Grilled Chicken Breast, Grilled Mahi-Mahi, and BBQ Grilled Shrimp are among the healthiest entrées on the menu, even trumping most of the salads.

Eat This

Cheese and Tomato Flatbread Pizza (individual)

and a House Side Salad with Fat-Free Vinaigrette

755 calories
30 g fat
(17 g saturated)
1,815 mg sodium

This pizza provides a whopping 85 percent of your daily allowance of saturated fat. But if you're going to Uno's in search of a slice, this is as good as it gets.

Other Picks

BBQ Grilled Shrimp	260 calories 2 g fat (0 g saturated) 1,000 mg sodium
7 oz. Filet Mignon	300 calories 12 g fat (4 g saturated) 440 mg sodium
Chicken Lettuce Wraps	390 calories 21 fat (3 g saturated) 960 mg sodium

Not That!

Chicago Classic Deep Dish Pizza (individual)

2,310 calories
162 g fat
(48 g saturated)
4,200 mg sodium

A horrific 228 percent of your daily allowance of fat and 167 percent of your daily sodium intake.

"Best Food Around." Order o... www.unos...

Other Passes

BBQ Chicken Flatbread Pizza
(individual)

810 calories
30 g fat (13.5 g saturated)
1,740 mg sodium

Steak Fajitas

920 calories
88 g fat (32 g saturated)
1,700 mg sodium

Pizza Skins

2,400 calories
155 g fat (50 g saturated)
600 mg sodium

GUILTY PLEASURE

Mediterranean Flatbread Pizza

690 calories
36 g fat (12 g saturated)
1,860 mg sodium

The spinach and tomatoes balance blood sugar, and eating whole olives, like the Kalamata variety on this pizza, provides fiber, vitamin E, and cancer-fighting phytochemicals.

MENU DECODER

● **SLUSH:** This neon drink on the kids menu is straight sugar, made entirely of red and blue cotton candy syrup (high-fructose corn syrup) poured over ice.

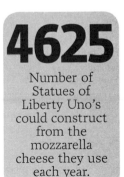

4625

Number of Statues of Liberty Uno's could construct from the mozzarella cheese they use each year.

Wendy's

● Wendy's is responsible for two popular innovations that have served to vastly increase the amount of fast food we as a nation consume: the introduction of the drive-thru window in 1970, and the birth of the Value Menu in 1988. Now, more than 40 percent of Americans claim to eat behind the wheel.

● Wendy's burgers were recently rated #1 in the fast food world by Zagat, the venerable restaurant rating guide. The fact that their beef is never frozen may account for this distinction.

Eat This

Ultimate Chicken Grill Sandwich

with Side Salad with Reduced Fat Creamy Ranch and Medium Iced Tea

540 calories
22 g fat
(4.5 g saturated)
1,780 mg sodium

The Ultimate Chicken Grill sandwich is the healthiest sandwich on the menu, serving up a fillet with only 1.5 grams of fat. If you want your chicken spicy, it will be fried instead of grilled, tacking on another 9.5 fat grams.

Other Picks

Small Chili and 5 Piece Crispy Chicken Nuggets

450 calories
21 g fat (5 g saturated)
1,300 mg sodium

Single with Everything

430 calories
20 g fat (7 g saturated)
900 mg sodium

Sour Cream & Chives Potato

320 calories
4 g fat (2.5 g saturated)
55 mg sodium

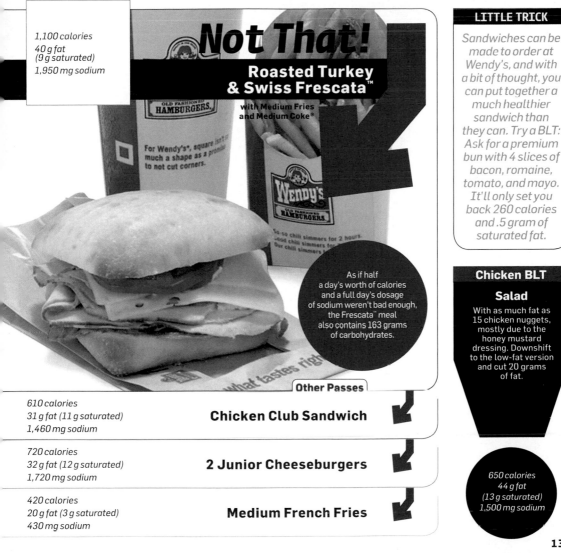

1,100 calories
40 g fat
(9 g saturated)
1,950 mg sodium

Not That!

Roasted Turkey & Swiss Frescata™

with Medium Fries and Medium Coke®

For Wendy's®, square isn't much a shape as a promise to not cut corners.

As if half a day's worth of calories and a full day's dosage of sodium weren't bad enough, the Frescata™ meal also contains 163 grams of carbohydrates.

LITTLE TRICK

Sandwiches can be made to order at Wendy's, and with a bit of thought, you can put together a much healthier sandwich than they can. Try a BLT: Ask for a premium bun with 4 slices of bacon, romaine, tomato, and mayo. It'll only set you back 260 calories and .5 gram of saturated fat.

Chicken BLT
Salad

With as much fat as 15 chicken nuggets, mostly due to the honey mustard dressing. Downshift to the low-fat version and cut 20 grams of fat.

650 calories
44 g fat
(13 g saturated)
1,500 mg sodium

Other Passes

610 calories
31 g fat (11 g saturated)
1,460 mg sodium

Chicken Club Sandwich

720 calories
32 g fat (12 g saturated)
1,720 mg sodium

2 Junior Cheeseburgers

420 calories
20 g fat (3 g saturated)
430 mg sodium

Medium French Fries

137

Chapter 3

MENU DECODER

Breakfast Diner

HOME FRIES

The breakfast equivalent of French fries, it's like waking up on the wrong side of the nutritional bed. The carb boost might give you an initial surge of energy, but you'll be running on empty long before lunch.

EGGS BENEDICT

Made from melted butter and egg yolks, the hollandaise that covers it is like a big blanket of cholesterol. Waiters don't like to serve this because they're afraid you won't live long enough to tip.

PANCAKES

These are usually made from white flour, whole milk, and eggs, for a total of 165 calories and 5 grams of fat apiece (before butter and syrup). A typical waffle has 550 calories and 21 grams of fat; a slice of French toast has 150 calories and 7 grams of fat.

SPINACH & FETA CHEESE OMELETTE

One of the most nutritious omelettes on the menu. Feta cheese has one-third less fat than cheddar (9.5 grams per ounce), and spinach is packed with nutrients such as vitamins A and C.

๛๛๛๛ BREAKFAST SPECIALS ๛๛๛๛

Our value-oriented breakfast specials come with your choice of coffee or tea and a small juice.
Add two eggs to any breakfast for $1.50.

MT. AIRY
TWO EGGS, ANY STYLE, 7.95
with your choice of breakfast meat, home fries, grits or white cheddar grits. White, wheat or rye toast.

Add Bagel or English muffin for $.50.

WAYNE JUNCTION
CLASSIC EGGS BENEDICT 8.95
Grilled Canadian bacon served under poached eggs and rich Hollandaise neatly stacked on a toasted English muffin. Comes with your choice of home fries, grits or white cheddar grits.

WYNDMOOR
THREE THICK-CUT SLICES OF CINNAMON-RAISIN CHALLAH FRENCH TOAST 7.95
with your choice of breakfast meat. Served dusted with powdered sugar.

GRAVERS
THREE FLUFFY BUTTERMILK PANCAKES 7.45
with your choice of breakfast meat.

Add bananas, blueberries or strawberries for 1.00

UPSAL
GOLDEN MALTED BELGIAN WAFFLE 7.45
with your choice of breakfast meat.

Add bananas, blueberries or strawberries and whipped cream for 1.00

ST. MARTIN'S
THREE HONEY-BUCKWHEAT PANCAKES 8.50
filled with bananas and served with your choice of breakfast meat.

Add blueberries or chocolate chips for 1.00

SEDGWICK
TEXAS-STYLE FRENCH TOAST 7.45
Three slices with your choice of breakfast meat. Served dusted with powdered sugar.

STENTON
TRADITIONAL FISH AND GRITS 8.95
featuring fried cornmeal-dusted catfish and white cheddar grits. Served with two eggs and your choice of white, wheat or rye toast.

TULPEHOCKEN
CORNED BEEF HASH WITH TWO EGGS ANY STYLE 8.50
with white, wheat or rye toast and your choice of home fries, grits or white cheddar grits.

QUEEN LANE
HOMEMADE CREAMED CHIPPED BEEF 7.95
over your choice of white, wheat or rye toast. Served with home fries, grits or cheese grits.

HEARTY HIGHLAND
PLAIN LOW-FAT YOGURT 7.45
with a cup of fresh fruit and granola.

๛๛๛๛ FROM THE GRIDDLE ๛๛๛๛

served with butter and syrup

Top your griddles with bananas, blueberries, chocolate chips or strawberry topping for 1.00
Add two eggs any style to your meal for 1.50   Add breakfast meat to any dish for 2.50

PANCAKES
FULL STACK (3)
SHORT STACK (2)

BUTTERMILK PANCAKES
Full Stack 4.25

[...] CAKES

CHOCOLATE CHIP PANCAKES
Full Stack 5.25
Short Stack 4.50

HONEY BUCKWHEAT PANCAKES
Full Stack 5.50
Short Stack 4.75

WHOLE GRAIN PANCAKES
Full Stack 5.50
Short Stack 4.75

FRENCH TOAST
TEXAS STYLE FRENCH TOAST
Full Stack 3.50
Short Stack 2.75

with Two Eggs, Any Style 4.75

BELGIAN WAFFLE
BELGIAN WAFFLE 3.50
with Fruit Topping 4.50

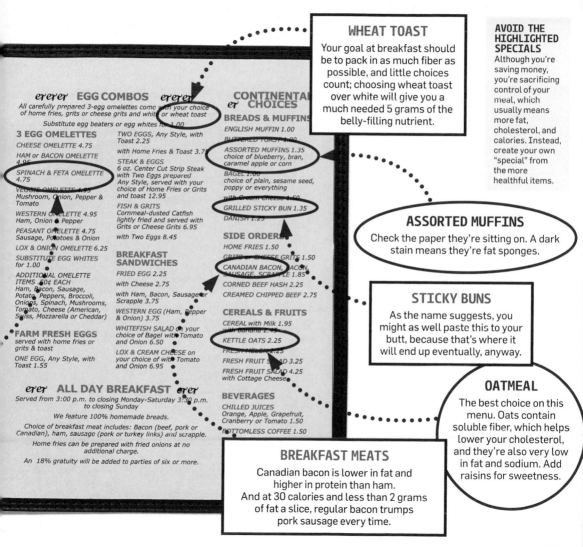

AVOID THE HIGHLIGHTED SPECIALS
Although you're saving money, you're sacrificing control of your meal, which usually means more fat, cholesterol, and calories. Instead, create your own "special" from the more healthful items.

WHEAT TOAST
Your goal at breakfast should be to pack in as much fiber as possible, and little choices count; choosing wheat toast over white will give you a much needed 5 grams of the belly-filling nutrient.

ASSORTED MUFFINS
Check the paper they're sitting on. A dark stain means they're fat sponges.

STICKY BUNS
As the name suggests, you might as well paste this to your butt, because that's where it will end up eventually, anyway.

OATMEAL
The best choice on this menu. Oats contain soluble fiber, which helps lower your cholesterol, and they're also very low in fat and sodium. Add raisins for sweetness.

BREAKFAST MEATS
Canadian bacon is lower in fat and higher in protein than ham. And at 30 calories and less than 2 grams of fat a slice, regular bacon trumps pork sausage every time.

EGG COMBOS

All carefully prepared 3-egg omelettes come with your choice of home fries, grits or cheese grits and white or wheat toast.
Substitute egg beaters or egg whites for 1.00

3 EGG OMELETTES

CHEESE OMELETTE 4.75

HAM or BACON OMELETTE 4.95

SPINACH & FETA OMELETTE 4.75

VEGGIE OMELETTE 4.95
Mushroom, Onion, Pepper & Tomato

WESTERN OMELETTE 4.95
Ham, Onion & Pepper

PEASANT OMELETTE 4.75
Sausage, Potatoes & Onion

LOX & ONION OMELETTE 6.25

SUBSTITUTE EGG WHITES for 1.00

ADDITIONAL OMELETTE ITEMS .50¢ EACH
Ham, Bacon, Sausage, Potato, Peppers, Broccoli, Onions, Spinach, Mushrooms, Tomato, Cheese (American, Swiss, Mozzarella or Cheddar)

FARM FRESH EGGS
served with home fries or grits & toast

ONE EGG, Any Style, with Toast 1.55

TWO EGGS, Any Style, with Toast 2.25

with Home Fries & Toast 3.75

STEAK & EGGS
6 oz. Center Cut Strip Steak with Two Eggs prepared Any Style, served with your choice of Home Fries or Grits and toast 12.95

FISH & GRITS
Cornmeal-dusted Catfish lightly fried and served with Grits or Cheese Grits 6.95

with Two Eggs 8.45

BREAKFAST SANDWICHES

FRIED EGG 2.25

with Cheese 2.75

with Ham, Bacon, Sausage or Scrapple 3.75

WESTERN EGG (Ham, Pepper & Onion) 3.75

WHITEFISH SALAD on your choice of Bagel with Tomato and Onion 6.50

LOX & CREAM CHEESE on your choice of with Tomato and Onion 6.95

ALL DAY BREAKFAST
Served from 3:00 p.m. to closing Monday-Saturday 3:30 p.m. to closing Sunday

We feature 100% homemade breads.

Choice of breakfast meat includes: Bacon (beef, pork or Canadian), ham, sausage (pork or turkey links) and scrapple.

Home fries can be prepared with fried onions at no additional charge.

An 18% gratuity will be added to parties of six or more.

CONTINENTAL CHOICES

BREADS & MUFFINS

ENGLISH MUFFIN 1.00

BUTTERED TOAST 1.00

ASSORTED MUFFINS 1.35
choice of blueberry, bran, caramel apple or corn

BAGEL 1.00
choice of plain, sesame seed, poppy or everything

with Cream Cheese 1.50

GRILLED STICKY BUN 1.35

DANISH 1.25

SIDE ORDERS

HOME FRIES 1.50

GRITS or CHEESE GRITS 1.50

CANADIAN BACON, BACON, SAUSAGE, SCRAPPLE 1.85

CORNED BEEF HASH 2.25

CREAMED CHIPPED BEEF 2.75

CEREALS & FRUITS

CEREAL with Milk 1.95
with Banana 2.45

KETTLE OATS 2.25

FRESH MELON 2.25

FRESH FRUIT SALAD 3.25

FRESH FRUIT SALAD 4.25
with Cottage Cheese

BEVERAGES

CHILLED JUICES
Orange, Apple, Grapefruit, Cranberry or Tomato 1.50

BOTTOMLESS COFFEE 1.50

Pizzeria

PIZZA An average slice of cheese pizza contains about 300 calories and 11 grams of fat, so order a side salad to keep from overindulging. A good way to reduce fat is to ask for part-skim mozzarella, which will save you up to 24 grams of fat on an entire pie. Avoid the most destructive toppings: pepperoni, sausage, ground beef, and extra cheese.

APPETIZERS

Most of these involve a vat of hot oil. Split an antipasto salad with the table instead: it's loaded with high-quality protein.

WHITE PIZZA AND PIZZA MARINARA

The two extremes of the pizza spectrum: one (marinara) has no cheese, and the other (white) has no sauce. The marinara is the better choice because that red sauce is packed with vitamins and very few calories. Try it. You'll be surprised how little you miss the cheese. On the other hand, white pizza (no tomato sauce) is like the Beatles with two Ringos and no John: more cheese, less substance.

FRESH GARLIC TOPPING

One-half to 1 clove of garlic a day has been shown to decrease total cholesterol.

Our PIZZA Pies

The "Drexel Hill" Jano
Our most popular pizza! Loaded with 7 toppings, it's one heavy pie! ~Sausage, Pepperoni, Mushrooms, Onions, Roasted Peppers, Black Olives and Extra Cheese! **16.59**

Meat Lovers Pizza
5 toppings ~ Bacon, Beef, Ham, Pepperoni, and Sausage **15.99**

The Cheese Steak Pizza
Topped with Fresh Grilled Rib Eye Steak, Mushrooms and Onions **15.59**

Veggie Pizza
A mountain of fresh vegetables are piled high onto our red pie **15.59**

Hawaiian Style Pizza
A red pie topped with tender diced ham & juicy pineapple chunks **12.99**

Buffalo Chicken
A red pie topped with tender cooked chicken breast, marinated in our own special buffalo sauce. **13.59**

The Upside Down
A combination of Provolone and Mozzarella cheese with sauce on top **11.59**

Red or White Pie
Red, Our version of the traditional Neapolitan, cheese pizza.
White, A delicious blend of fresh garlic, oregano, Ramano, Mozzarella, and our special white herb sauce! **9.59**

Pizza Marinara
No Cheese, vegan option! **8.59**

Appetizers & Sides

Mozzarella Sticks
Six lightly seasoned breaded mozzarella sticks w/ marinara sauce. **6.29**

Chicken Fingers
5 Breaded chicken breast tenderloins, fried to golden brown perfection, served w/ BBQ sauce, or tossed in buffalo sauce & served w/ blue cheese dressing. **6.79**

Chicken Finger Platter
Same as Chicken Fingers above, but with French Fries **8.99**

Buffalo Wings
Tender Chicken wings, golden fried, then tossed in buffalo sauce. Served w/ blue cheese dressing. **(24) 12.49**

Cheese Fries
A large order of fries, smothered in cheese sauce **3.79**

Pizza Fries
A large order of fries, lightly covered with pizza sauce and smothered with oven melted mozzarella. **3.99**

French Fries
A large order of our delicious golden fries. **3.29**

Onion Rings
A large order of our golden battered onion rings. **3.99**

Garlic Bread
One of our 12" french rolls covered with fresh garlic & toasted. **2.99**

Old World Salads

Antipasto Salad

Quality Italian meats & cheese over a bed of romaine lettuce topped with olives, onions, roasted peppers, shredded parmesan & red wine vinaigrette **8.50**

Grilled Chicken Salad

Lightly seasoned, grilled chicken breast on top of our house salad. **8.50**

Buffalo Chicken Salad

Breaded chicken tenderloin strips, tossed in buffalo sauce, on top of our house salad. **8.50**

Caesar Salad

Fresh chopped Romaine lettuce, croutons, black olives, and shredded parmesan cheese with Caesar dressing served on the side **6.50**

House Salad

Fresh chopped Romaine lettuce, red onions, black olives & tomatoes. with blue cheese, ranch or red wine vinaigrette **5.50**

Hoagies & Grinders

Hoagies: A cold submarine type sandwich with Provolone or white american cheese, your choice of meats & topped with iceberg lettuce, Roma tomatoes, oil & vinegar, and pepper and oregano sprinkled on top. Mayo, mustard, red onions, black olives, sweet peppers, or anything else, upon request (additional charges may apply)

Grinders: Your choice of meats, topped with white american, mozzarella, or provolone, and oven toasted to melt the cheese and give the roll that perfect crusty crunch, then topped with iceberg lettuce, fresh sliced Roma tomatoes, oil & vinegar, pepper and oregano sprinkled on top.

The Old School Italian

A prime selection of Ham, Procuitto, Salami, & spicy Cappacola with Provolone Cheese **7.49**

Italian

Ham, Salami, spicy Cappacola and Provolone **6.99**

Turkey Breast **6.99**

Ham & Cheese **6.99**

Albacore Tuna **6.99**

Italian Specialty Grinders:

Chicken Parmesan Sandwich

Golden fried breaded chicken tenderloins, sliced and stuffed inside our 12" rolls, topped with marinara, and mozzarella or provolone cheese and oven toasted **6.99**

Eggplant Parmesan Sandwich **6.99**

Create Your Own Pasta

Choose your pasta: Spaghetti, penne, or fusilli.

Choose your sauce: Alfredo, tomato, pesto, or clam. **6.99**

ITALIAN HOAGIE

Generally contains the fattiest lunch meats, including beef salami (12 grams of fat per serving), capicola (16 grams) and pepperoni (24 grams). That's 52 grams of fat, not counting the oil and cheese! By contrast, turkey breast contains 1/12 the fat of the beef salami.

PARMESAN

The fastest way to ruin a lean protein or defenseless vegetable? Bread it, fry it, and smother it in cheese. An eggplant alone only has 60 calories, but by the time it's done getting parm-ed, it has 1,000 calories and 68 grams of fat.

SAUCE DECODER

PASTA SAUCES

Listed in ascending order of destructiveness:

Tomato

Virtually fat-free, plus cooked tomatoes are a proven prostate protector.

Pesto

High in fat, but most of that is healthy monounsaturated fat from olive oil. Plus basil and garlic both contain cancer-fighting compounds.

Clam

The simple rule: Red is good; white is bad.

Alfredo

Butter, cream, and cheese on the pasta amount to 860 calories and 45 grams of fat per 2-cup serving.

Mexican Cantina

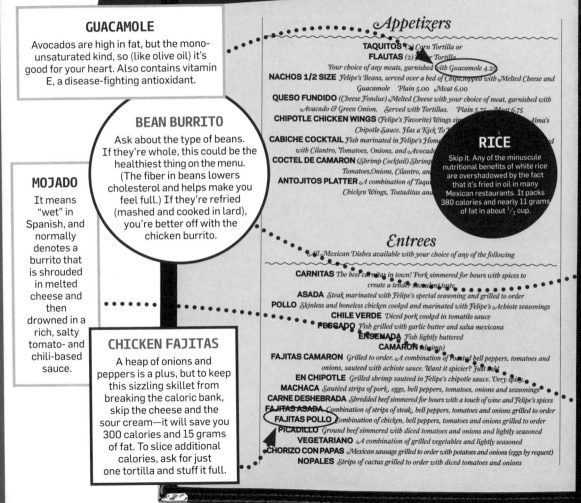

GUACAMOLE
Avocados are high in fat, but the mono-unsaturated kind, so (like olive oil) it's good for your heart. Also contains vitamin E, a disease-fighting antioxidant.

BEAN BURRITO
Ask about the type of beans. If they're whole, this could be the healthiest thing on the menu. (The fiber in beans lowers cholesterol and helps make you feel full.) If they're refried (mashed and cooked in lard), you're better off with the chicken burrito.

MOJADO
It means "wet" in Spanish, and normally denotes a burrito that is shrouded in melted cheese and then drowned in a rich, salty tomato- and chili-based sauce.

RICE
Skip it. Any of the minuscule nutritional benefits of white rice are overshadowed by the fact that it's fried in oil in many Mexican restaurants. It packs 380 calories and nearly 11 grams of fat in about $1/2$ cup.

CHICKEN FAJITAS
A heap of onions and peppers is a plus, but to keep this sizzling skillet from breaking the caloric bank, skip the cheese and the sour cream—it will save you 300 calories and 15 grams of fat. To slice additional calories, ask for just one tortilla and stuff it full.

Appetizers

TAQUITOS (3) Corn Tortilla or
FLAUTAS (2) Flour Tortilla
Your choice of any meats, garnished with Guacamole 4.25
NACHOS 1/2 SIZE Felipe's Beans, served over a bed of Chips, topped with Melted Cheese and Guacamole   Plain 5.00   Meat 6.00
QUESO FUNDIDO (Cheese Fondue) Melted Cheese with your choice of meat, garnished with Avocado & Green Onion.   Served with Tortillas.   Plain 5.75   Meat 6.75
CHIPOTLE CHICKEN WINGS (Felipe's Favorite) Wings sim... ...Alma's Chipotle Sauce. Has a Kick To I...
CABICHE COCKTAIL Fish marinated in Felipe's Hom... with Cilantro, Tomatoes, Onions, and Avocado...
COCTEL DE CAMARON (Shrimp Cocktail) Shrimp... Tomatoes, Onions, Cilantro, an...
ANTOJITOS PLATTER A combination of Taqui... Chicken Wings, Tostaditas and...

Entrees
All Mexican Dishes available with your choice of any of the following

CARNITAS The best carnitas in town! Pork simmered for hours with spices to create a tender, succulent taste.
ASADA Steak marinated with Felipe's special seasoning and grilled to order
POLLO Skinless and boneless chicken cooked and marinated with Felipe's Achiote seasonings
CHILE VERDE Diced pork cooked in tomatilo sauce
PESCADO Fish grilled with garlic butter and salsa mexicana
ENSENADA Fish lightly battered
CAMARON (shrimp)
FAJITAS CAMARON Grilled to order. A combination of roasted bell peppers, tomatoes and onions, sauteed with achiote sauce. Want it spicier? Just ask!
EN CHIPOTLE Grilled shrimp sauteed in Felipe's chipotle sauce. Very spicy.
MACHACA Sautéed strips of pork, eggs, bell peppers, tomatoes, onions and seasonings
CARNE DESHEBRADA Shredded beef simmered for hours with a touch of wine and Felipe's spices
FAJITAS ASADA Combination of strips of steak, bell peppers, tomatoes and onions grilled to order
FAJITAS POLLO Combination of chicken, bell peppers, tomatoes and onions grilled to order
PICADILLO Ground beef simmered with diced tomatoes and onions and lightly seasoned
VEGETARIANO A combination of grilled vegetables and lightly seasoned
CHORIZO CON PAPAS Mexican sausage grilled to order with potatoes and onions (eggs by request)
NOPALES Strips of cactus grilled to order with diced tomatoes and onions

A La Carte

TACOS

All tacos are served on a soft flour tortilla with cheese and lettuce. Hard shell or corn tortilla by request.

Taco filled with...
- Asada, Fajitas Asada 3.50
- Carne Desbebrada, Carne Desbebrada, Carnitas, Pollo, Picadillo, Fajitas Pollo, Chorizo con Papas, Nopales, Machacha, Chile Verde 3.25
- Ensenada or Pescado 3.50
- Camaron 4.75

TACO SALAD

Lettuce, rice, beans, jack and cheddar cheese, fresh salsa, guacamole, sour cream served with or without crisp shell

BURRITOS

A meal in itself that starts with a large flour tortilla and your choice of any meat, then we add rice, beans and cheese all wrapped inside. Frijoles de la olla by request.

Burrito filled with...
- Asada, Fajitas Asada, Chile Relleno 8.00
- Carne Desbebrada, Carnitas, Pollo, Picadillo, Fajitas Pollo, Vegetariano, Chorizo con Papas,
- Nopales, Machaca, Chile Verde 7.25
- Ensenada or Pescado 8.50
- Camaron 9.50

BURRITO MOJADO

A flour tortilla filled with your choice of meat and beans

topped with lettuce, tomato, cheese, and your choice of red or green salsa.

BURRITO AMERICANO

Grilled steak or chicken, smothered with Glazed Onions and garnished with Romaine Lettuce, Tomatoes, Cheese, Sliced Avocados & Felipe's sauce, all wrapped in a Tortilla. 7.25

- Chimichanga style, Enchilada, or Ranchero Style, or any other sauce add 2.00

TOSTADAS

A crisp corn tortilla spread with beans, your choice of entree, topped with fresh lettuce, guacamole sauce and cheese.

Tostadas with...
- Asada, Fajitas Asada 8.00
- Carne Desbebrada, Carnitas, Pollo, Picadillo, Fajitas Pollo, Vegetariano 7.25

NACHOS

First we start with a layer of beans, add a good portion of fresh chips, add more beans, your favorite meat and cover it with melted cheese and garnished with guacamole sauce.

Nachos with...
- Asada, Fajitas Asada 8.50
- Carne Desbebrada, Carnitas, Pollo, Picadillo 7.50

QUESADILLAS

Your choice of meat and melted cheese in between two flour tortillas, garnished with guacamole.

Quesadillas with...
- Asada 8.00
- Carne Desbebrada, Carnitas, Pollo, Picadillo 7.45
- Camarones (Shrimp) of your choice 10.25

TAQUITOS AND FLAUTAS

Our homemade taquitos are made with corn tortillas and our flautas are made with flour tortillas, topped with guacamole & lettuce.

ENCHILADAS

A soft corn tortilla, stuffed with cheese or meat, and smothered with enchilada sauce or tomatillo sauce then topped with melted cheese and lettuce.

Enchiladas with...
- Carne Desbebrada, Carnitas, Pollo 4.25
- Cheese 4.25
- Camaron 4.75

CHILE RELLENO

A Chile Poblano stuffed with cheese and topped with special sauce.

MOLE

Mexico's national mole dish. A blend of ancho chiles, almonds, peanuts and filberts. Served with chicken.

TACO ON A SOFT FLOUR TORTILLA

Lower in fat than a hard shell tortilla. But don't go loco: A large tortilla can pack more than 250 calories. For an even better option, ask them to make your tacos with corn tortillas; every Mexican restaurant has them on hand to make enchiladas, and they'll cut another 100 calories from each taco, plus add a few grams of fiber.

TACO SALAD

It's a huge fried tortilla shell with ground beef, cheese, sour cream, and a few token shreds of iceberg lettuce. The result: 900 calories, 55 grams of fat, and perhaps the most liberal use of the word "salad" ever.

ENCHILADAS

Typically, these tortillas are dipped in hot fat, stuffed, rolled, covered with sauce and cheese, and baked. When topped with sour cream, two of them carry 748 calories, 55 percent of which comes from fat.

MOLE

A complex sauce containing up to 40 ingredients, including chilies, ground nuts, spices, and often chocolate. Smothering grilled chicken or enchiladas, it's a vast nutritional improvement on melted cheese and sour cream.

Sports Bar

NACHOS
Fresh tortilla chips topped with melted cheddar cheese, chili, black olives, tomatoes, onions, sour cream, and jalapeños. $8.85

CHICKEN TENDERS
Tender white meat, breaded and deep fried until golden brown. $8.85

POTATO SKINS
Potato skins topped with melted cheddar cheese, real bacon bits, and green onions. Served with sour cream. $7.85

BUFFALO WINGS
Thick, meaty chicken wings, celery and carrots. You choose hot, mild, teriyaki or Randy Jones BBQ flavor. Served with ranch or blue cheese for dipping. $8.85

HOG WINGS
Tender, juicy pork that peels off the bone covered in BBQ Sauce. $8.85

POPCORN CHICKEN
Bite-sized pieces of breaded chicken. $7.85

SHRIMP BASKET
Breaded shrimp, served with cocktail sauce. 7.85

FRIED CALAMARI
Tubes and tentacles lightly breaded, served with a house special cajun ranch dip. $7.85

CHEESE STICKS
Melted, breaded mozzarella cheese sticks served with ranch dip or marinara sauce. $8.85

BEEF BURGER
Wood-Fired Beef Burger served with Lettuce, Tomato $7.85

POTATO SKINS
Best relative choice among the appetizers, as long as they're baked, not fried. (Fried ones have 420 calories and 40 grams of fat *per skin* if stuffed with cheese and topped with sour cream.)

BEER A bad beer choice could cost you 100 calories a bottle. For the healthiest light beers, sip Miller® Lite, Michelob® ULTRA™, or Amstel® Light—all have less than 100 calories and 5 grams of carbohydrates. Want a full-flavored beer? Try Guinness® Draught, with only 126 calories in a 12-ounce bottle.

BEEF BURGER
The difference between a hamburger with ketchup, mustard, and produce and a cheeseburger with mayo is 250 calories and 20 grams of fat. You can have the burger, as long as you show some restraint.

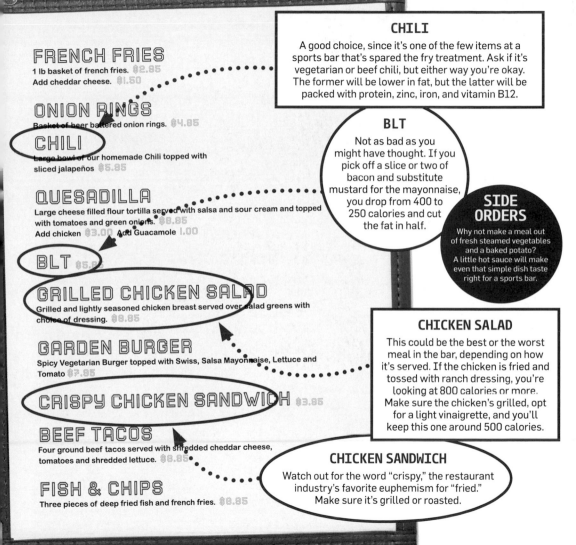

FRENCH FRIES
1 lb basket of french fries. $2.95
Add cheddar cheese. $1.50

ONION RINGS
Basket of beer battered onion rings. $4.95

CHILI
Large bowl of our homemade Chili topped with
sliced jalapeños $5.95

QUESADILLA
Large cheese filled flour tortilla served with salsa and sour cream and topped
with tomatoes and green onions. $8.95
Add chicken $3.00 Add Guacamole 1.00

BLT $5.95

GRILLED CHICKEN SALAD
Grilled and lightly seasoned chicken breast served over salad greens with
choice of dressing. $9.95

GARDEN BURGER
Spicy Vegetarian Burger topped with Swiss, Salsa Mayonnaise, Lettuce and
Tomato $7.95

CRISPY CHICKEN SANDWICH $3.95

BEEF TACOS
Four ground beef tacos served with shredded cheddar cheese,
tomatoes and shredded lettuce. $8.95

FISH & CHIPS
Three pieces of deep fried fish and french fries. $8.95

CHILI
A good choice, since it's one of the few items at a
sports bar that's spared the fry treatment. Ask if it's
vegetarian or beef chili, but either way you're okay.
The former will be lower in fat, but the latter will be
packed with protein, zinc, iron, and vitamin B12.

BLT
Not as bad as you
might have thought. If you
pick off a slice or two of
bacon and substitute
mustard for the mayonnaise,
you drop from 400 to
250 calories and cut
the fat in half.

SIDE ORDERS
Why not make a meal out
of fresh steamed vegetables
and a baked potato?
A little hot sauce will make
even that simple dish taste
right for a sports bar.

CHICKEN SALAD
This could be the best or the worst
meal in the bar, depending on how
it's served. If the chicken is fried and
tossed with ranch dressing, you're
looking at 800 calories or more.
Make sure the chicken's grilled, opt
for a light vinaigrette, and you'll
keep this one around 500 calories.

CHICKEN SANDWICH
Watch out for the word "crispy," the restaurant
industry's favorite euphemism for "fried."
Make sure it's grilled or roasted.

Sushi

Appetizers

House Salad
Edamame
Avocado Salad
Spicy Tako Salad
Spicy Shrimp Salad
Ika Sansai
Seaweed Salad
Yakitori (chicken, beef, pork, seafood)

Roll Appetizer (3pcs Californ roll, 3pcs crab salad roll, 3pcs takka maki, 3pcs negi hamach
Sashimi Appetizer Combo (tuna, white fish & octopus)
Sushi Appetizer Combo (nigiri: tuna, white fish, shrim crabstick & 2 pcs tekka maki)
Sunomono (choice of: crab, octopus or shrimp)

EDAMAME

High in protein and fiber and very low in calories, steamed soybeans make a good start to a meal. Cooks tend to dust them heavily in salt before sending them to your table; ask the server for your edamame salt-less, and apply it carefully yourself.

YAKITORI

Skewers of lean meat and vegetables give you maximum nutrition for minimum calories. Couldn't be a better start to a meal: protein- and nutrient-packed and grilled over an open flame.

Specialty Rolls

Black & White (white fish tempura, scallions, black sesame seeds & seaweed)
Buddy Buddy (tuna, hamachi & wasabi tobiko topped with fresh salmon & ikura)
Grand Canyon (unagi, avocado & cucumber topped with broiled white tuna, masago & silver sauce)
Green Dragon (Alaska king crab, unagi & tempura crunch with avocado)
Hawaiian (spicy salmon, tempura crunch & cucumber topped with avocado & tuna)
Jumbo (crabstick, cucumber, hamachi, unagi & masago

Fire Island (California roll & tempura crunch topped with spicy tuna & scallions)
Fuji Volcano (shrimp tempur topped with unagi & spicy masago sauce)
Matsu (unagi, avocado, crabstick, tamago & masago
Rainbow (California roll toppe with tuna, white fish, smoked salmon, shrimp & hamachi)
Snow Mountain (shrimp tempura & cucumber topped with Alaska king crab & masag
Tekka Tuna (spicy tuna, tempura crunch topped with tuna sashimi)

CALIFORNIA ROLL

The most popular menu item is also one of the most healthy. Just 300 calories for eight pieces, plus a dose of healthy fat from the avocado.

Hand Roll Special

3 handrolls
One tuna, one yellowtail & one crab salad roll
Cooked Sushi Combo
Pieces of nigiri to include: shrimp, octopus, crab stick, tamago, smoked salmon & a crab salad roll
Chirashi
Assorted Sashimi on a bed of sushi rice

Rolls Rolls Rolls
Three pices of each: Tekka mak negi hamachi maki, California roll, Mexican roll, Alaska roll, Philadelphiaroll and 4 pieces of futomaki
Deluxe Sashimi
9 pcs each: fresh salmon, hamachi, white fish, tako & 2 pc kani & tamago
Omakase
Chef's choice of Sashimi

SOY SAUCE

Japanese sushi purists scoff when they see Westerners drowning their fish in puddles of soy muddied with a mound of wasabi. They should: A single tablespoon of soy sauce has over 1,000 mg of sodium. At a reputable sushi spot, the chef will serve the fish exactly as it's intended to be eaten, which means hands off the soy.

HOUSE SALAD

Sounds healthy, right? The iceberg it's served on offers very little nutritionally, and 2 tablespoons of the oily ginger dressing can have up to 200 calories and 10 grams of fat. Branch out and try the seaweed salad, one of nature's most potent multivitamins, instead.

Don Buri

Sashimi on a bed of sushi rice served with House Salad & Miso Sou

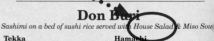

Tekka
Ikura

Hamachi
Fresh Salmon

Sushi Combinations
Served with Miso Soup & Salad

Matsu Sushi Dinner
California roll, spicy tekka maki, 5pcs nigiri sushi consisting of: tuna, shrimp, white fish, tamago and smoked salmon

Traditional Sushi & Sashimi Dinner Traditional Sushi Dinner plus sashimi appetizer

Traditional Sushi Dinner
Nigiri sushi consisting of: tuna, white fish, mackeral, smoked salmon, yellowtail, shrimp, octopus, crab stick, tamago, crab roe & tekka maki

Nigiri-Sushi
One serving consists of two pieces

Alaska King Crab
Amaebi (sweet shrimp)
Blue Fin Tuna
Ebi (boiled shrimp)
Escolar (seared fatty white tuna)
Hamachi (yellowtail)
Hirame (fluke)
Hotategai (scallop)
Hokkigai (surf clam)
Ika (squid)
Ikura (salmon roe)
Kanikama (crab stick)
Kanpachi (wild yellowtail)
Masago (crab roe)
Saba (spanish mackerel)

Shake (fresh salmon)
Shake (smoked salmon)
Spicy Tuna (original or jalapeno)
Spicy scallop (original or jalapeno)
Suzuki (bass)
Tai (red snapper)
Tako (boiled octopus)
Tarako (cod roe)
Tamago (layered chicken eggs)
Tobiko (flying fish roe)
Unagi (fresh water eel)
Uni (sea urchin)
Wakame (seaweed)
Quail egg

Maki Sushi
One serving consists of 6 pieces unless noted

Alaska Roll (smoked salmon, cream cheese & masago)
California Roll (crab stick & cucumber)
Crab Salad Roll
Futomaki 4 pcs (crab stick, shrimp, tamago, pickle & cucumber)
Gobo Maki (pickled burdock)
Ikura Maki (salmon roe)
Kampo Maki (oriental squash)
Kappa Maki
Mexican Roll (boiled shrimp & avocado)
Negi Hamachi Maki (yellowtail & scallions)
Natto Maki (fermented soybeans)

Philadelphia Roll (smoked salmon, cream cheese & masago)
Sake Kawa Maki (smoked salmon skin & cucumber)
Shrimp Tempura Maki 4 pcs (shrimp tempura, cucumber & crab roe)
Spicy Scallop Maki (original or jalapeno)
Spicy Tekka Maki (spicy tuna original or jalapeno)
Spider Maki 4 pcs (soft shell crab roll & masago)
Takuwan Maki (pickled radish)
Tekka Maki (tuna roll)
Unagi Maki (fresh water eel)
Ume Maki 2 pcs (plum paste & oba leaf)

NIGIRI / SASHIMI
The Japanese live longer than anyone on the planet. The reason? Fish. Nigiri is individual pieces of fish draped over rice; sashimi is just pieces of raw fish. Save yourself the unnecessary carbohydrates and go straight for the plain fish.

TOBIKO
The Japanese word for flying fish eggs. A tablespoon of the neon-colored stuff has about 20 percent of your daily cholesterol in it. Limit yourself to one tobiko-strewn item per sushi session.

SPANISH MACKEREL
Oft-overlooked for more glamorous fish like salmon and tuna, the humble mackerel has twice the amount of heart-healthy, inflammation-reducing, cancer-fighting omega-3 fatty acids as salmon, making it one of the healthiest fish in the sea.

SPICY TUNA ROLL
The "spicy" comes from a dab of Asian chili sauce mixed with mayo. Bad. Want something fiery? Ask for chili sauce on the side, or an extra mound of wasabi.

BBQ Joint

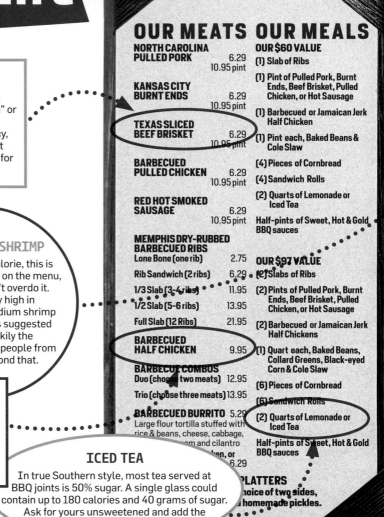

OUR MEATS

NORTH CAROLINA PULLED PORK	6.29
	10.95 pint
KANSAS CITY BURNT ENDS	6.29
	10.95 pint
TEXAS SLICED BEEF BRISKET	6.29
	10.95 pint
BARBECUED PULLED CHICKEN	6.29
	10.95 pint
RED HOT SMOKED SAUSAGE	6.29
	10.95 pint

MEMPHIS DRY-RUBBED BARBECUED RIBS

Lone Bone (one rib)	2.75
Rib Sandwich (2 ribs)	6.29
1/3 Slab (3–4 ribs)	11.95
1/2 Slab (5–6 ribs)	13.95
Full Slab (12 Ribs)	21.95

BARBECUED HALF CHICKEN	9.95

BARBECUE COMBOS

Duo (choose two meats)	12.95
Trio (choose three meats)	13.95

BARBECUED BURRITO	5.29

Large flour tortilla stuffed with rice & beans, cheese, cabbage, ... m and cilantro ... ken, or
... 6.29

PLATTERS
...hoice of two sides, ... homemade pickles.

OUR MEALS

OUR $60 VALUE

(1) Slab of Ribs

(1) Pint of Pulled Pork, Burnt Ends, Beef Brisket, Pulled Chicken, or Hot Sausage

(1) Barbecued or Jamaican Jerk Half Chicken

(1) Pint each, Baked Beans & Cole Slaw

(4) Pieces of Cornbread

(4) Sandwich Rolls

(2) Quarts of Lemonade or Iced Tea

Half-pints of Sweet, Hot & Gold BBQ sauces

OUR $97 VALUE

(2) Slabs of Ribs

(2) Pints of Pulled Pork, Burnt Ends, Beef Brisket, Pulled Chicken, or Hot Sausage

(2) Barbecued or Jamaican Jerk Half Chickens

(1) Quart each, Baked Beans, Collard Greens, Black-eyed Corn & Cole Slaw

(6) Pieces of Cornbread

(6) Sandwich Rolls

(2) Quarts of Lemonade or Iced Tea

Half-pints of Sweet, Hot & Gold BBQ sauces

BEEF BRISKET

They'll ask you if you prefer your brisket "lean" or "moist." Opt for the former—it's plenty juicy, and in this case, moist is merely a euphemism for "riddled with fat."

PEEL 'N' EAT SHRIMP

Fat-free and low-calorie, this is the healthiest starter on the menu, as long as you don't overdo it. Shrimp are very high in cholesterol—10 medium shrimp have 30% of a day's suggested intake—but luckily the shell-peeling keeps people from going much beyond that.

CHICKEN

The leanest meat on the menu by a healthy margin. Opt for the smoked or rotisserie chicken over the greasy fried stuff and keep the calorie count around 500.

ICED TEA

In true Southern style, most tea served at BBQ joints is 50% sugar. A single glass could contain up to 180 calories and 40 grams of sugar. Ask for yours unsweetened and add the sugar (carefully) yourself.

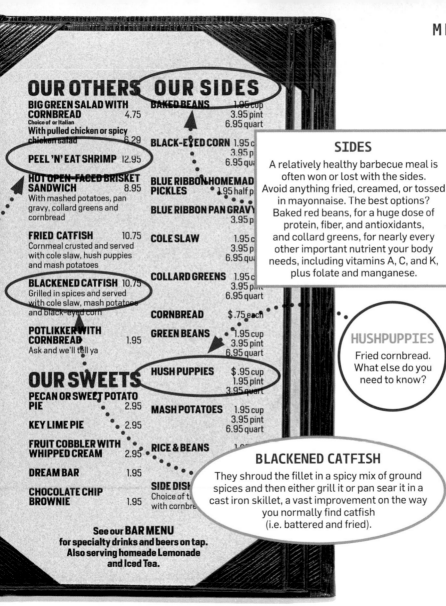

OUR OTHERS

BIG GREEN SALAD WITH CORNBREAD 4.75
Choice of or Italian

With pulled chicken or spicy chicken salad 6.29

PEEL 'N' EAT SHRIMP 12.95

HOT OPEN-FACED BRISKET SANDWICH 8.95
With mashed potatoes, pan gravy, collard greens and cornbread

FRIED CATFISH 10.75
Cornmeal crusted and served with cole slaw, hush puppies and mash potatoes

BLACKENED CATFISH 10.75
Grilled in spices and served with cole slaw, mash potatoes and black-eyed corn

POTLIKKER WITH CORNBREAD 1.95
Ask and we'll tell ya

OUR SWEETS

PECAN OR SWEET POTATO PIE 2.95

KEY LIME PIE 2.95

FRUIT COBBLER WITH WHIPPED CREAM 2.95

DREAM BAR 1.95

CHOCOLATE CHIP BROWNIE 1.95

See our BAR MENU
for specialty drinks and beers on tap.
Also serving homeade Lemonade
and Iced Tea.

OUR SIDES

BAKED BEANS 1.95 cup
3.95 pint
6.95 quart

BLACK-EYED CORN 1.95 cup
3.95 pint
6.95 quart

BLUE RIBBON HOMEMADE PICKLES 1.95 half pint

BLUE RIBBON PAN GRAVY 3.95 pint

COLE SLAW 1.95 cup
3.95 pint
6.95 quart

COLLARD GREENS 1.95 cup
3.95 pint
6.95 quart

CORNBREAD $.75 each

GREEN BEANS 1.95 cup
3.95 pint
6.95 quart

HUSH PUPPIES $.95 cup
1.95 pint
3.95 quart

MASH POTATOES 1.95 cup
3.95 pint
6.95 quart

RICE & BEANS 1.95

SIDE DISH
Choice of t...
with cornbre...

SIDES

A relatively healthy barbecue meal is often won or lost with the sides. Avoid anything fried, creamed, or tossed in mayonnaise. The best options? Baked red beans, for a huge dose of protein, fiber, and antioxidants, and collard greens, for nearly every other important nutrient your body needs, including vitamins A, C, and K, plus folate and manganese.

HUSHPUPPIES

Fried cornbread. What else do you need to know?

BLACKENED CATFISH

They shroud the fillet in a spicy mix of ground spices and then either grill it or pan sear it in a cast iron skillet, a vast improvement on the way you normally find catfish (i.e. battered and fried).

CLIFF NOTES

RIBS

With different cuts, sauces, and dry rubs to consider, proper rib ordering requires its own manual. Here are the Cliff Notes:

Kansas City Spare Ribs
Kansas City–style 'cue is usually heavily sauced, which can mean a huge dose of sugar from the barbecue sauce.

Memphis-Style Baby Back Ribs
Cut from the upper section of the loin, baby backs are the leanest rib you'll find at a BBQ joint. Try to get them dry rubbed, if possible: You'll save the calories from the sauce, plus you'll actually be able to taste the meat, and not just a mouthful of sauce.

St. Louis Spare Ribs
Cut from the belly, aka the bacon zone. The fattiest of all standard rib cuts.

Texas-Style Ribs
Very fatty; the only redeeming quality of these ribs is that they're usually smoked with just salt and pepper, rather than the sugary barbecue sauces found on other ribs.

Steakhouse

Appetizers

Smoked Pacific Salmon

Maine Lobster Cocktail

Jumbo Lump Crabmeat Cocktail

Broiled Sea Scallops Wrapped in Bacon, Apricot Chutney

Colossal Shrimp Cocktail

Oysters on the Half Shell

Jumbo Lump Crab Cake

Colossal Shrimp Alexander

Lobster Bisque

Tuna Tartare

DRY AGED

High-end butchers and steakhouses hang meat for up to 45 days to allow excess moisture to evaporate and to break down tough muscle fibers, leaving a more intensely flavored, tender piece of beef. The process can be very expensive, and because they only use fatty, well-marbled steaks for dry aging, it will hurt you in the wallet *and* in the gut.

ICEBERG WEDGE SALAD

Combine the least nutritious of all salad leaves, iceberg, with a fatty, salty blue cheese dressing, and you're left with a 400+-calorie starter with no real redeeming qualities. The better option is the mixed green or the tomato-and-onion salads.

Salads

Center Cut Iceberg

Caesar Salad

Morton's Salad

Sliced Beefsteak Tomato, Purple Onion, Vinaigrette or Blue Cheese

Chopped Salad

VEGETABLES

Grilled asparagus and steamed vegetables are two of the only items on the steakhouse menu that don't contribute to your waistline. Forget creamed spinach—it can carry up to 400 calories and 20 grams of fat in a small scoop.

Vegetables & Potatoes

Steamed Fresh Jumbo Asparagus, Sauce Hollandaise

Grilled Jumbo Asparagus, Balsamic Glaze Steamed Fresh Broccoli

Creamed Spinach

Sauteed Fresh Spinach & Mushrooms

Jumbo Baked Idaho Potato

Lyonnaise Potatoes

Mashed Potatoes

Potato Skins

Sauteed Wild Mushrooms

Sauteed Onions

POTATOES

Baked naked or mashed. Every other option—hash browns, fries, potato gratin—turn the simple spud into a sponge for fat.

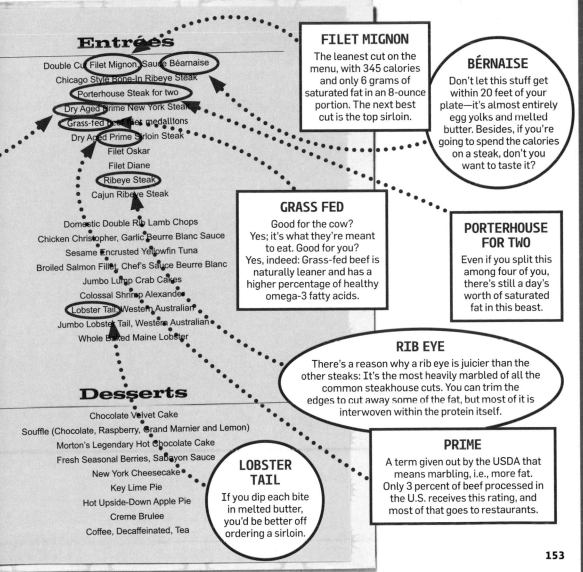

Entrées

Double Cut Filet Mignon, Sauce Béarnaise
Chicago Style Bone-In Ribeye Steak
Porterhouse Steak for two
Dry Aged Prime New York Steak
Grass-fed beef filet medallions
Dry Aged Prime Sirloin Steak
Filet Oskar
Filet Diane
Ribeye Steak
Cajun Ribeye Steak

Domestic Double Rib Lamb Chops
Chicken Christopher, Garlic Beurre Blanc Sauce
Sesame Encrusted Yellowfin Tuna
Broiled Salmon Fillet, Chef's Sauce Beurre Blanc
Jumbo Lump Crab Cakes
Colossal Shrimp Alexander
Lobster Tail, Western Australian
Jumbo Lobster Tail, Western Australian
Whole Baked Maine Lobster

Desserts

Chocolate Velvet Cake
Souffle (Chocolate, Raspberry, Grand Marnier and Lemon)
Morton's Legendary Hot Chocolate Cake
Fresh Seasonal Berries, Sabayon Sauce
New York Cheesecake
Key Lime Pie
Hot Upside-Down Apple Pie
Creme Brulee
Coffee, Decaffeinated, Tea

FILET MIGNON
The leanest cut on the menu, with 345 calories and only 6 grams of saturated fat in an 8-ounce portion. The next best cut is the top sirloin.

BÉRNAISE
Don't let this stuff get within 20 feet of your plate—it's almost entirely egg yolks and melted butter. Besides, if you're going to spend the calories on a steak, don't you want to taste it?

GRASS FED
Good for the cow? Yes; it's what they're meant to eat. Good for you? Yes, indeed: Grass-fed beef is naturally leaner and has a higher percentage of healthy omega-3 fatty acids.

PORTERHOUSE FOR TWO
Even if you split this among four of you, there's still a day's worth of saturated fat in this beast.

RIB EYE
There's a reason why a rib eye is juicier than the other steaks: It's the most heavily marbled of all the common steakhouse cuts. You can trim the edges to cut away some of the fat, but most of it is interwoven within the protein itself.

PRIME
A term given out by the USDA that means marbling, i.e., more fat. Only 3 percent of beef processed in the U.S. receives this rating, and most of that goes to restaurants.

LOBSTER TAIL
If you dip each bite in melted butter, you'd be better off ordering a sirloin.

Indian

SAMOSAS

These are small turnovers stuffed, most commonly with mashed potatoes, then fried. Add 200 calories a pop, they're not an ideal start to a meal.

PAKORA

Yes, they're vegetables, in theory. But they're battered and deep-fried before they hit the plate, which means they pick up a lot of excess baggage on the way to your mouth.

SOUP

Since so many of the appetizers in Indian cuisine revolve around potatoes and the deep fryer, start your meal with a bowl of soup instead. Indian soups are broth-based and packed with vegetables, which means plenty of nutrients and a scarcity of calories.

NAAN

The crispy charred flatbread can be more addictive than chips and salsa before a Mexican meal. Share an order with the table and have them bring it out with the meal: You'll need it to sop up the fragrant sauces.

APPETIZERS

VEGETABLE SAMOSA Two crisp turnovers, stuffed with delicately spiced potatoes, peas, and herbs. $2.50

VEGETABLE PAKORA Assorted vegetable fritters gently seasoned and deep fried. $2.50

CHICKEN PAKORA Chicken fritters, deep fried. $3.25

SHRIMP PAKORA Shrimp dipped in spiced batter, deep fried. $5.95

HOUSE SPECIAL PLATTER A fine presentation of our choice appetizers, recommended for two. $6.95

VEGETARIAN PLATTER Assorted vegetable appetizers, recommended for two. $5.95

PANEER PAKORA Pieces of homemade cheese, dipped in chickpea flour and fried. $3.25

SOUPS AND SALADS

VEGETABLE SOUP Soup made from fresh vegetable, lentils, spices and flavored with delicate herbs. $2.50

MULLIGATAWNY SOUP A traditional chicken soup with lentils and spices. $2.50

COCONUT SOUP A soup with fresh milk and coconut, served hot with pistachios. $2.50

RAITA Homemade whipped yoghurt with cucumbers, potatoes and fresh mint leaves. 2.50

GREEN SALAD Lettuce, tomatoes, green peppers, and onions. $2.50

BREADS

NAAN Leavened fine flour bread, soft and fluffy. $2.25

PARATHA Whole wheat bread, butter layered $2.25

ROTI Whole wheat bread $1.50

ALOO PARATHA Whole wheat bread, stuffed with potatoes $2.50

PANEER KULCHA Naan stuffed with homemade cheese, spices and herbs $2.50

KEEMA NAAN Fine flour bread, stuffed with ground lamb, fresh ginger, and cilantro $2.95

POORI Whole wheat puffy bread, deep fried in vegetable oil $2.95

CHICKEN CURRIES

CHICKEN CURRY The original cooked in onions, garlic, ginger, yoghurt, and spices $9.95

CHICKEN MAKHANI The legendary tandoori chicken, masterfully cooked in tomato and garlic sauce $10.95

CHICKEN SHAHI KORMA Tender chicken delicately cooked in a rich sauce with nuts and cream $9.95

CHICKEN SAAGWALA Boneless chicken cooked with creamed spinach $9.95

CHICKEN TIKKA MUGLAI Tandoori chicken and mushrooms cooked in tomato and garlic sauce $10.95

CHICKEN TIKKA BHUNA Chicken tikka cooked dry with browned onions, tomato and bell peppers $9.95

CHICKEN TIKKA MASALA Tandoori roasted chicken tikka, in a tomato and butter sauce $10.95

CHICKEN JALFEREZI Tender, boneless chicken cooked with spring onions,tomato and bell peppers $9.95

CHICKEN DILRUBA Chicken cooked with mushrooms $9.95

CHICKEN ASPARAGUS Chicken cooked with asparagus and fresh spices sauce $10.95

CHICKEN ACHAR Chicken cooked in tomato onion, gravy with pickled spices $9.95

CHICKEN CHILLY Tendar boneless chicken pieces, onions, tomatoes, bell peppers cooked in sweet and sour sauce, mint flavored (Mild, med. or hot) $10.95

CHICKEN VINDALOO Boneless chicken and potatoes in a highly spiced sauce $9.95

VEGETABLE CURRIES

SAAG PANEER Chunks of homemade cheese in creamed spinach and fresh spices $8.95

ALOO SAAG Spinach and potatoes with fresh spices $8.95

NAVRATAN CURRY Nine assorted garden fresh vegetables sauteed in a traditional onion and tomato sauce $8.95

ALOO GOBHI MASALA Fresh cauliflower and potatoes, cooked dry in onions, tomatoes and herbs $8.95

MATTAR PANEER Fresh homemade cheese, cooked gently with tender garden peas and fresh spices $8.95

ALOO MATTAR Garden fresh green peas and potatoes with fresh spices $8.95

MATTAR MUSHROOMS Garden fresh peas and mushroms cooked with garlic, ginger, and onions $8.95

BAIGAN BHARTHA Roasted eggplant sauteed in onion, tomatoes and green peas $8.95

DAL MAKHANI Black lentils and beans, cooked in onions, with tomatoes and cream $8.95

MALAI KOFTA KASHMIRI *Garden fresh vegetables and homemade cheeseballs cooked in a rich sauce with nuts and cream $9.95*

CHANNA MASALA PUNJABI *A North Indian specialty, subtly flavored chick peas, tempered with ginger $8.95*

KADI PAKORA SINDHI *Dumpling of mixed vegetables, cooked in chick peas flour, yoghurt and mustard sauce $8.95*

PANEER SHAHI KORMA *Tender chunks of homemade cheese, cooked with nuts and a touch of cream in fresh herbs and spices $9.95*

PANEER MASALA *Tender chunks of homemade cheese, cooked with tomato and butter sauce $9.95*

PANEER ACHAR *Homemade cheese cooked in tomato onion gravy with pickled spices $9.95*

PANEER CHILLY *Homemade cheese, onions, tomatoes, bell peppers cooked in sweet and sour sauce, mint flavored $9.95*

LAMB SHAHI KORMA *Tender lamb, in a rich sauce with nuts and cream $10.95*

LAMB SAAGWALA *Chunks of lamb in creamed spinach $10.95*

LAMB BHUNA *Pan-broiled lamb, cooked in specially prepared herbs and spices with a touch of ginger and garlic $10.95*

LAMB VINDALOO *Lamb and potatoes cooked in a sharply spiced tangy sauce $10.95*

KEMMA MATTAR *Ground lamb cooked with peas and herbs $10.95*

BOTI KABAB MASALA *Tandoor broiled lamb sauteed in our special exquisite curry to gastronomic satisfaction $11.95*

LAMB ACHAR *Tender lamb cooked in tomato, onion, gravy with pickled spices $10.95*

LAMB ASPARAGUS *Lamb and asparagus cooked in a special ginger, garlic and onion sauce $11.95*

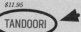

TANDOORI

TANDOORI CHICKEN *Chicken marinated in yoghurt and freshly ground spices, then broiled in the tandoor (half) $9.95*

CHICKEN TIKKA *Boneless, tender chicken, gently broiled $9.95*

RESHMI KABAB *Mild, tender, pieces of chicken breast, marinated in a very mild sauce, barbecued on a skewer in the tandoor $10.95*

BOTI KABAB *Juicy cubes from leg of lamb, broiled to perfection in the tandoor $10.95*

SEEK KABAB *Finger rolls of ground lamb, spiced with fresh ginger $10.95*

TANDOORI FISH *Swordfish marinated in an exotic recipe of exciting spices and herbs, broiled on charcoal $13.95*

TANDOORI SHRIMP *Jumbo shrimp seasoned with fresh spices and herbs, baked in the tandoor $14.95*

OUR CHEF RECOMMENDS

SEAFOOD FANTASY *Start with tandoori fish and tandoori shrimp, followed by your choice of shrimp masala or shrimp cury, dal, naan, pullao and green salad. $19.95*

THALI HOUSE VEGETARIAN *A traditional Indian meal served on a silver platter with dal, chanamasala, mattar paneer, rice, poori or roti, raita and gulab jamun. $12.95*

VEGETABLE SEEKHAM *Fresh carrots, cauliflower, green peas, homemade cheese, pineapple chunks cooked with spices, sauce and nuts. $9.95*

LAMB DANSHIK *Tender lamb and chick peas lentils cooked with pineapple chunks and herbs. $11.95*

LAMB KASHMIRI *Lamb cooked in an onion, ginger, garlic and peach sauce. $11.95*

CHICKEN LA-JAWAB *Tender boneless chicken pieces and apple chunks cooked in ginger, garlic sauce and nuts. $11.95*

RICE SPECIALTIES

VEGETABLE BIRYANI *A mulgai-inspired dish of curried rice with vegetables, dried fruits and nuts $8.95*

CHICKEN BIRYANI *Classic mulgai dish of curried rice with chicken, dried fruits and nuts $9.95*

LAMB BIRYANI *Curried rice with lamb, dried fruits and nuts $10.95*

SHRIMP BIRYANI *White shrimp and rice in dried fruits and nuts $11.95*

HOUSE SPECIAL BIRYANI *Our special biryani cooked with chicken, lamb, shrimp, vegetables, dried fruits and nuts $13.95*

PEAS PULLAO *Rice cooked with peas, raisins and nuts $3.95*

PLAIN RICE *$1.95*

VEGETARIAN

Indian chefs can do things with vegetables that you didn't think were possible. Stick to dishes based on lentils and chickpeas for protein, and mushrooms, spinach, and tomatoes for maximum nutrient intake.

TANDOORI

A great place to start on any Indian menu. Tandoori means cooked in a tandoor, a traditional clay oven that gets up to 900°F, India's incendiary answer to the grill. If available, try tandoori fish or shrimp—both make for delicious meals under 500 calories.

CHICKEN TIKKA

Lean chicken marinated in yogurt and spices, this makes an excellent entrée choice. But don't mistake chicken tikka with tikka masala; masala means "cream" in Hindi, and that means "fat" in any language.

DAL

Find a way to make these super-flavorful stewed lentils a part of your meal—they're an excellent low-fat source of protein and fiber.

LAMB

Lamb figures heavily into Indian cuisine, and most of it either comes from the shoulder or the leg, both of which contain a large portion of fat. Count on lamb entrées being 200 calories more than their chicken counterparts.

Tapas

Soups And Salads

SOPAS DEL DIA
Soups of the day — ask your server for today's choices **$6**

ENSALADA DE QUESOS DE CABRA
Four Goat Cheese Salad with sliced Pears, Toasted Pine Nuts, Baby Greens, and an Aged Balsamic Vinegar Reduction **$10**

ENSALADA DEL MONJE
Baby Spinach with imported Cabrales Blue Cheese, Toasted Pi... with an Aged Sherry Vinaigrette $9...

ENSALADA V...
Seasonal Baby Greens tossed with Champagne–Citru... Oregano Crouto...

ENSALADA MEDI...
Greens, Tomato, Hearts of Palm, Sweet Bell Pep... Bluefin Tuna Loin with White...

ENSALADA DE AGUACA...
...ts of Romaine, Carrots, Hearts of Palm, Avocado, ...made Brandy Dressing **$10**

Vegetables And Cheeses

ACEITUNAS Y ALMENDRAS
Assorted Marinated Olives & Marcona almonds **$4**

QUESO MAHÓN FRITO CON SALSA DE TOMATE
Fried Mahon Cheese with Spicy Tomato Sauce **$8**

QUESO IDIAZABAL CON TOMATE, ORÉGANO Y LCAPARRONES
Smoked Basque Idizabal Cheese with sliced Tomatoes, Fresh Oregano, and Caperberries **$10**

PIMIENTOS ASADOS EN CAZUELA CON QUESO DE CABRA
Marinated roasted Red and Yellow Bell Peppers with melted fresh Spanish Goat Cheese **$7**

PATATAS BRAVAS
Deep fried potatoes in a spicy sauce

BERENJENA FRITA AL SALMOREJO
Fried Eggplant with Salmorejo Sauce **$7** with Serrano Ham **$10**

PIMIENTOS DEL PIQUILLO AL AJILLO
Sauteed strips of roasted Piquillo Peppers with toasted Garlic slivers **$7**

PATATAS ALI-OLI
Fried Baby Red Potatoes with an unabashed Garlic Ali-oli **$6**

TORTILLA ESPAÑOLA
The Classic Potato and Onion Omelette from Spain **$8**

CROQUETAS
Breadcrumbs are wrapped around a filling made from a mix of flour, milk, butter, and cheese or ham, and then the whole package is deep-fried. Think: fat bomb.

ALMONDS AND OLIVES
Along with a glass of vino, this is a traditional start to a Spanish meal. And it's a good one: All three of the beloved Spanish staples help fight off cardio-vascular disease. No wonder Spaniards live longer than nearly everyone else on the planet.

MEDIAS RACIONES
Half portions, a standard serving size in the tapas world. Even if you're not into the whole plate-passing thing, there's good news: Flavor-packed small plates can be just as filling as larger portions, according to research from Cornell University.

SANGRIA
Can be sweetened with fruit, sugar, or both. Ask if they use sugar in their recipe. If so, you're better off ordering red wine.

PATATAS BRAVAS
Cubed, fried potatoes covered with garlic mayo and hot sauce. Want heat? Go with roasted piquillo peppers instead.

TORTILLA ESPAÑOLA
Ubiquitous staple of the tapas menu, this Spanish-style omelet gives paella a run for its money as the national dish. Made simply of egg, onion, and potato, it's a safe haven for confused and calorie-conscious diners alike.

Fish And Seafood

PAELLA DE MARISCOS
Prawns, mussels, squid, peppers, peas and onions served in a rich saffron rice. **$12**

PEZ EN ADOBO
Fresh Mahi-Mahi, cubed and marinated in the style of Cadiz, battered and perfectly fried **$7**

GAMBAS AL AJILLO
Sauteed Shrimp with sliced Garlic and Pequin Chile Flake served sizzling hot in a Cazuela **$7**

CALAMARES FRITOS CON DOS SALSAS
Flash fried Baby Calamari with Spicy Tomato Sauce and Roast Garlic Caper Ali-oli **$8**

VIEIRAS AL VINO BLANCO CON JAMÓN SERRANO
Sautéed Scallops with White Wine and Serrano Ham **$10**

CROQUETAS DE JAMÓN
Serrano Croquettes with Roast Garlic-Caper Alioli and Baby Greens **$7**

BOQUERONES EN ESCABECHE
Fresh white Anchovy filets marinated in Garlic and Parsley **$7**

MEJILLONES AL VINO CON TOMATE
Steamed cultured Mediterranean Black Mussels with herbed White Wine and Tomato Broth **$12**

VIERAS A LA GALLEGA
Baked Scallops in their own Shell with Galician Tomato, Paprika and White Wine Sauce topped with Bread Crumbs **$10**

Meat And Poultry

JAMÓN SERRANO
The famous mountain cured Ham of Spain, shaved to order **$12**

PINCHOS MORUNOS
Spicy marinated grilled Brochettes Lamb **$9** Chicken **$6**

CHORIZO A LA PARRILLA CON PESTO
Grilled Chorizo Sausage with Parsley and Pine Nut Pesto **$7**

CHAMPINONES RELLENOS DE CHORIZO
Broiled Mushroom Caps stuffed with Chorizo Sausage and topped with Manchego Cheese **8**

SPANISH MEAT & CHEESE PLATE
Chef's Selection of Spanish Cured Meats, Chorizo & Spanish Cheese **$4**

ALBÓNDIGAS A LA CORDOBESA
Braised Pork Meatballs in a Saffron Roast Chicken Broth **$6**

SOLOMILLO DE RES AL CABRALES
Grilled 3oz Filet Mignon with Blue Cheese Cream Sauce and Red Wine Carmelized Onions **$12**

PAELLA
Order the "*mariscos*" version whenever possible. It's traditional along the coast of Spain and includes a variety of clams, mussels, squid, and shrimp, much better than the chorizo and chicken thigh version that's also common.

GAMBAS AL AJILLO
Shrimp with a ton of garlic. A single order of these crustaceans might be sautéed in up to $1/4$ cup of olive oil, which is good for your heart, but ultimately packs nearly 500 calories on its own.

MUSSELS AND CLAMS
A good rule of thumb is to gravitate toward the shellfish. Whether steamed with white wine and herbs or served with a chunky tomato sauce, the protein fills you up while the shell negotiating slows you down. A portion won't cost you more than 400 calories.

MEAT AND CHEESE PLATE
A common option in Spanish restaurants. Meats are sliced super thin, so order wisely and this can be a solid beginning to a meal. Pick lean *lomo* and *jamón serrano* over fat-speckled chorizo.

Seafood

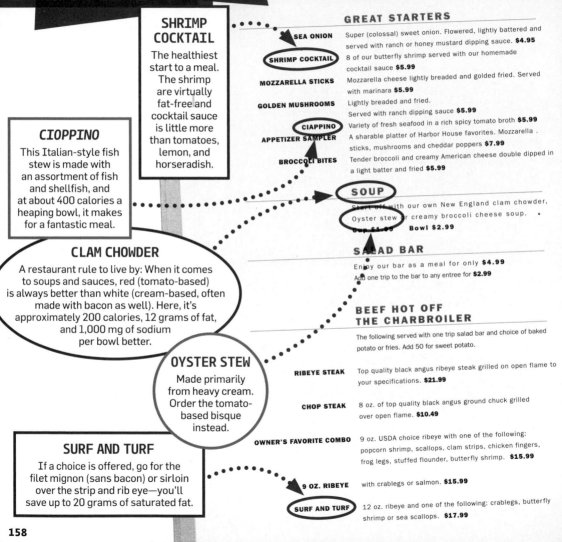

SHRIMP COCKTAIL

The healthiest start to a meal. The shrimp are virtually fat-free and cocktail sauce is little more than tomatoes, lemon, and horseradish.

CIOPPINO

This Italian-style fish stew is made with an assortment of fish and shellfish, and at about 400 calories a heaping bowl, it makes for a fantastic meal.

CLAM CHOWDER

A restaurant rule to live by: When it comes to soups and sauces, red (tomato-based) is always better than white (cream-based, often made with bacon as well). Here, it's approximately 200 calories, 12 grams of fat, and 1,000 mg of sodium per bowl better.

OYSTER STEW

Made primarily from heavy cream. Order the tomato-based bisque instead.

SURF AND TURF

If a choice is offered, go for the filet mignon (sans bacon) or sirloin over the strip and rib eye—you'll save up to 20 grams of saturated fat.

GREAT STARTERS

SEA ONION — Super (colossal) sweet onion. Flowered, lightly battered and served with ranch or honey mustard dipping sauce. **$4.95**

SHRIMP COCKTAIL — 8 of our butterfly shrimp served with our homemade cocktail sauce **$5.99**

MOZZARELLA STICKS — Mozzarella cheese lightly breaded and golded fried. Served with marinara **$5.99**

GOLDEN MUSHROOMS — Lightly breaded and fried. Served with ranch dipping sauce **$5.99**

CIAPPINO — Variety of fresh seafood in a rich spicy tomato broth **$5.99**

APPETIZER SAMPLER — A sharable platter of Harbor House favorites. Mozzarella sticks, mushrooms and cheddar poppers **$7.99**

BROCCOLI BITES — Tender broccoli and creamy American cheese double dipped in a light batter and fried **$5.99**

SOUP

Start off with our own New England clam chowder, Oyster stew or creamy broccoli cheese soup. •
Cup $1.99   **Bowl $2.99**

SALAD BAR

Enjoy our bar as a meal for only **$4.99**
Add one trip to the bar to any entree for **$2.99**

BEEF HOT OFF THE CHARBROILER

The following served with one trip salad bar and choice of baked potato or fries. Add 50 for sweet potato.

RIBEYE STEAK — Top quality black angus ribeye steak grilled on open flame to your specifications. **$21.99**

CHOP STEAK — 8 oz. of top quality black angus ground chuck grilled over open flame. **$10.49**

OWNER'S FAVORITE COMBO — 9 oz. USDA choice ribeye with one of the following: popcorn shrimp, scallops, clam strips, chicken fingers, frog legs, stuffed flounder, butterfly shrimp. **$15.99**

9 OZ. RIBEYE — with crablegs or salmon. **$15.99**

SURF AND TURF — 12 oz. ribeye and one of the following: crablegs, butterfly shrimp or sea scallops. **$17.99**

FRIED SEAFOOD

DAILY SPECIAL	Served with slaw, hushpuppies and choice of baked potato or fries. Add 50 for sweet potato.
HARBOR HOUSE SPECIAL	Alaskan whitefish, butterfly shrimp, oysters, sea scallops, devil crab and clam strips all fried golden brown and served with slaw, hushpuppies and choice of baked potato or fries. Add 50 for sweet potato. This platter not available broiled.
MONDAY	2 pc whitefish & popcorn shrimp $7.99
TUESDAY	2 pc chicken tender & popcorn shrimp $7.99
WEDNESDAY	2 pc flounder & popcorn shrimp **$7.99**
THURSDAY	Regular popcorn shrimp platter **$7.99**
	Large popcorn shrimp platter **$9.49**
FRIDAY & SATURDAY	Ask your server

POPCORN SHRIMP, CRAB CAKES & FRIED OYSTERS

Think of the fryer as the great equalizer: It turns everything that touches it into nutritional garbage. Whenever possible, take your oysters raw, your shrimp steamed, and your crab cakes—well, just leave that one alone.

FRIED PLATTERS

Served with slaw, hushpuppies and tartar sauce.

Fish & Popcorn Shrimp 10.49
Popcorn Shrimp 7.99
Clam Strips 7.99
Skinless, Boneless Flounder 7.99
Skinless, Boneless Grouper 7.99
Farm Raised Catfish Filets 7.99
Sea Scallops 13.99
Oysters 13.99
Butterfly Shrimp 12.99

TARTAR SAUCE

Nutritionally bankrupt dipping sauce, with up to 10 grams of fat in a single tablespoon. Opt for fat-free cocktail sauce, made mostly of tomatoes and horseradish or, better yet, a squeeze of lemon.

OVEN BROILED SEAFOOD

BROILED FISH	Choose from Alaskan whitefish, Flounder or Catfish. Boneless, skinless, broiled in our special seasonings. Served over rice pilaf. **$10.99**
SWORDFISH	a thick steak covered in herb butter and broiled. Served over rice pilaf. **$12.99**
GRILLED ATLANTIC SALMON	An 8 oz. portion of delicious pink salmon seasoned and grilled over an open flame. Served over rice pilaf. **$10.99**
BLACKENED AHI TUNA	with ginger-citrus sticky rice, sesame sugar snaps, sweet soy and wasabi **$22.99**
BUTTERFLY SHRIMP	12 pieces of shrimp basted in our unique mixture of seasonings, then broiled. Served over rice pilaf. **$14.99**
SCALLOPS	Fresh sea scallops perfectly seasoned and broiled. Served over rice pilaf. **$15.99**

SWORDFISH

Along with shark and king mackerel, this meaty fish has been shown to have dangerously high mercury levels. Skip it altogether. Shrimp, salmon, albacore tuna, and catfish are all excellent, lower-mercury options, especially important for pregnant women and children.

BLACKENED

It means covered in a piquant blend of spices—paprika, onion powder, and cumin—and cooked on high heat, most often in a cast iron skillet. Blackening is a great, healthy way to add big flavor to dishes without excess calories.

Chinese

SEASAME/ORANGE/GENERAL TSO'S

The unholy trinity of crispy chicken dishes. Could you pick these three out of a lineup? Probably not. That's because each one is fried, then covered, vegetable-less, with gloppy, sugar-laden sauces almost indistinguishable from each other. The damage: About 1,300 calories and 70 grams of fat.

SOUP

Start your meals at Chinese restaurants with soup, either egg drop or hot and sour. They have a mere 70 calories per cup and will help blunt any of the ravenous hunger that leads to overeating.

ENTRÉES Here's a ratio worth forgetting at Chinese restaurants: 1 entrée to 1 diner. At over a pound (and usually 1,000 calories) per order, these heaping plates and overstuffed cartons are really meant to serve two. If it's variety you seek, order one per person, but ask them to bring half out and box the other half for lunch tomorrow.

STEAMED

The optimal word on a Chinese menu. Seek it out aggressively and make sure at least one item you order has this word in the name or in the menu description.

FORTUNE COOKIE

The most innocuous dessert you'll find in any restaurant: Each little cookie has a mere 40 calories.

APPETIZERS

	Pu Pu Platter (for 2)	$7.25
	Egg Rolls, Chicken Fingers, Spareribs, Teriyaki Chicken Wings, Crab Rangoon	
	...Fingers	$7.25
	...Platter	$9.95
	...Beef (2), Boneless Spare Ribs, Chicken	
	...Crab Rangoon (2), Chicken Teriyaki (2)	
	...Spareribs	$7.25
	...Teriyaki (6)	$7.55
	...Rangoon (6)	$4.25
	Egg Roll (2)	$3.75
A13.	Dim Sim Siu Mi (6)	$4.75
A5.	Shanghai Spring Rolls (2)	$3.95
A14.	Chicken Teriyaki	$7.55
A15.	Vegetable Egg Rolls(2)	$3.95
A7.	Chicken Wings (7)	$5.95
A8.	Fried Shrimps (6)	$7.55
A17.	Scallion Pancake	$3.95
A9.	Spareribs	$7.55
A18.	Dumplings (Pork or Vegetable) (6)	$3.95

SOUP

S1.	Wonton Soup	$2.05
S5.*	Hot and Sour Soup	$2.05
S2.	Egg Drop Soup	$1.65
S6.	Chinese Vegetable Soup	$2.05
S3.	House Special Soup	$7.55

BEEF

B1.	Beef with Green Peppers	$9.55
B10.	Beef with Mushrooms	$10.25
B2.	Beef with Broccoli	$9.55
B11.*	Beef in Szechuan Sauce	$9.55
B3.	Beef with Pea Pods	$9.55
B12.*	Spicy Beef with Peanuts and Hot Peppers	$9.55
B4.	Crispy Beef with Pea Pods	$9.55
B13.*	Spicy Shredded Beef in Garlic Sauce	$9.55
B5.	Beef with Pea Pods and Bamboo Shoots	$10.25
B14.*	Hunan Spiced Beef	$9.55
B6.	Mongolian Barbecued Beef	$10.25
B15.*	Beef with Black Bean Sauce	$9.55
B7.	Beef with Scallions	$9.55
B16.*	Orange Flavored Beef	$10.55
B8.	Beef with Chinese Vegetables	
B17.*	House Special Lamb	
B9.	Sesame Beef	

* Hot & Spic   Fortune Cookies offered by C

HINT

Always use chopsticks, especially if you're bad with them. Not because it's culturally correct, but because it makes you work for your food; the longer it takes us to bring the food from plate to lips, the more time we give our stomach to deliver the time-delayed message of "I'm full, please stop" to our brains.

LUNCH

Served daily 11:30 a.m. to 2:30 p.m. (except Sunday & choice of Hot and Sour Soup, Egg Drop Sou

1.	Chicken Wings (3), Egg Roll	$5.2
12.*	Spicy Chicken with Peanuts, Spareribs	$5.5
2.	Teriyaki Beef (2), Chicken Wings (2), Egg Roll	$5.9
13.	Eight Treasure Chicken, Teriyaki Beef	$6.7
3.	Boneless Spareribs (4), Egg Roll	$5.9
14.	Chicken with Pea Pods, Chicken Fingers (3)	$6.2
4.	Teriyaki Beef (2), Spareribs (2), Shrimp (2)	$6.9
15.*	General Tso's Chicken, Egg Roll	$7.2
9.	Chicken Fingers (4), Chicken Wings (2)	$5.5
16.	Combo Lo Mein, Boneless Spareribs	$5.7
6.	Sweet and Sour Pork, Egg Roll	$5.2
17.*	Shrimp with Garlic Sauce, Egg Roll	$7.2

AUTHENTIC

Serv

W1.	Moo Goo Gai Pan	$5.0
W6.*	Szechuan Spicy Bean Curd (Meatless)	$4.8
W2.*	Chicken with Vegetables in Szechuan Sauce	$5.0
W7.	Beef with Vegetables in Oyster Sauce	$5.8
W3.	Chicken with Broccoli	$5.0

PORK

P1.	Pork with Pea Pods	$8.95
P5.*	Spicy Double Cooked Pork	$8.95
P2.	Pork with Broccoli	$8.95
P6.*	Spicy Shredded Pork in Garlic Sauce	$8.95
P3.	Pork with Scallions	$8.95
		$8.95
P4.	Three Delights with Pork, Shrimp, or Chicken	$9.55

POULTRY

C1.	Chicken with Cashews	$9.05
	Chicken	$9.05
	...ods	$9.05
	...Bean Sauce	$9.05
		$9.75
		$9.05
		$9.05
		$9.05

****

ECIALS

with choice of Pork Fried Rice or Steamed Rice and
(Soup not included with Take-Out orders).

Sweet and Sour Chicken, Egg Roll	$5.25
. Shrimp with Lobster Sauce, Egg Roll	$7.25
Beef with Green Pepper, Egg Roll	$6.25
.* Szechuan String Beans, Egg Roll	$5.35
Beef with Broccoli, Chicken Finger	$6.25
ii. Vegetarian's Delight, Egg Roll	$5.95
.* Spicy Double Cooked Pork, Egg Roll	$5.55
.* Meatless Chow Mein, Egg Roll	$4.25
(Or choice of Chicken, Shrimp, Beef or Pork Chow	
Mein)	$4.55
ii. Pork with Broccoli, Egg Roll	$5.75
2.* Shredded Beef Szechuan Style (Or choice of	
Chicken, Shrimp, or Pork	$4.55

SE LUNCH

Rice

3.* String Beans with Shredded Beef	$5.80
4.* Spicy Szechuan Beef With Peanuts	$5.70
9.* Broccoli in Garlic Sauce	$4.80
5.* Baby Shrimp with Peanuts	$5.70
40. Fried Bean Curd with Vegetables	$4.80

****

16.*	Jordan Chicken (General Gau's Chicken)	$9.75
17.*	Chef's Chicken Delight with Spicy Sesame	$9.95
6.	Chicken with Pineapple	$9.05
7.*	Spicy Szechuan Chicken with Peanuts	$9.05
18.*	Sesame Crispy Chicken	$9.95
19.*	Fresh String Beans with Chicken and Beef	$9.05
8.*	Spicy Shredded Chicken in Garlic Sauce	$9.05
20.*	Crispy Lemon Chicken	$9.95
9.*	Hunan Chicken with Black Mushrooms and Broccoli	$9.05
10.*	Chicken and Beef Hunan Style	$11.55

WEIGHT WATCHERS

All Weight-Watchers' orders are steamed. There is no
seasoning or corn starch used in cooking.

#1.	Mixed Vegetables	$5.95
#2.	Mixed Vegetables (Choice of Pork, Chicken, Beef or Shrimp)	$8.95
#3.	Broccoli or Snow Pea Pods or Asparagus	$5.95

MOO-SHI

Moo-Shi is a very popular mandarin dish which
mushrooms, cabbage, fungus, dried lily flower,
meat served with 6 pancakes and Hoi Sin

MI.	Moo-Shi (Chicken, Beef, Pork, Shrimp, or Vegetables)	
M2.	Moo-Shi Peking Style (Spicy)	

VEGETABLES

V1.	Vegetarian's Delight	$6.55
V5.	Stir Fried Pea Pods	$6.55
V6.*	Spicy Eggplant in Garlic Sauce	$6.25
V3.	Snow Pea Pods with Water Chestnuts	$6.55
V7.*	Spicy Broccoli	$6.25
V4.	Brocoli in Oyster Sauce	$6.55
V8.*	String Beans, Szechuan Style (Meatless)	$6.25

SWEET AND SOUR

SW1.	Sweet and Sour Pork	$7.55
SW3.	Sweet and Sour Shrimp	$8.95
SW2.	Sweet and Sour Chicken	$7.55
SW4.	Sweet and Sour Combo	$9.55

DUCK

Served with pancakes, scallions and Hoi Sin sauce

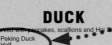

D1.	Peking Duck	
	Half	$14.00
	Whole	$27.00
D2.	Chef's Special Duck	
	Half	$13.00
	Whole	$25.00

NOODLES

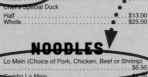

L1.	Lo Mein (Choice of Pork, Chicken, Beef or Shrimp)	$6.95
L2.	Combo Lo Mein	$7.25
L4.	Shanghai Noodles	$9.25
L6.	Shanghai Noodles (Meatless)	$6.95
L7.	Cold Noodles in Sesame Sauce	$4.95

RICE

R1.	Steamed Rice	$0.9
R2.	Fried Rice (Choice of Pork, Chicken, Beef)	$5
R3.	Combo Fried Rice	$7
R6.	Brown Rice	$1.5

SWEET AND SOUR

A surefire cue that something has been deep-fried and
covered in a sickly-sweet pink sauce.
Eat with rice and you're looking at a 1,000-calorie meal.

PEKING DUCK

Most of the fat from the skin
renders out of the duck over the
course of cooking, making
this a healthier option than most
of the stir-fry entrées available.
Order a side of steamed
vegetables and serve it with
a small scoop of
brown rice.

LO MEIN

Seems innocent enough,
right? But the noodles are
wok-fried with an abundance of
oil, then speckled with fatty
pork or beef. Even ordering
the vegetable version won't
undo the wrong wrought by
this dish. Stay away.

RICE

Keep rice consumption to a minimum:
A single portion can cost you 300 calories. Order
brown rice whenever possible. It won't save
you calories, fat, or carbohydrates, but it will give
you an extra boost of fiber and protein,
which work to boost metabolism and
keep you feeling full.

French Bistro

ONION SOUP

It's onions, broth, and very little else, which makes it a good starter, as long as you hold off on the floating crouton covered in Gruyère cheese that normally accompanies this soup.

SOUPS

6 ~~Soupe Du Jour~~
6 French Onion Soup
8 ~~Soupe D'Haricot~~
PURÉE OF HARICOT VERTS

BEURRE BLANC

A relative of Hollandaise, a few meager tablespoons of this butter-based sauce add hundreds of calories to whatever they touch.

APPETIZERS

7
Grilled Yellow Tuna Niçoise Salad
TUNA, HARICOT VERTS, BABY CARROTS, OLIVES, PEAR TOMATOES

5
Salade Parisienne
MIXED GREEN SALAD WITH HAM, SWISS CHEESE, ARTICHOKE HEARTS, CHERRY TOMATOES AND BOILED EGGS IN A CITRUS HERB VINAIGRETTE DRESSING

TUNA NIÇOISE

The very best thing you can order at a bistro. The tuna packs on the protein and the omega-3 fatty acids, while the A-list roster of vegetables (tomatoes, green beans, peppers) bring a heap of nutrients and powerful antioxidants to the salad.

6
Tomato Mozzarella Salad
FRESH TOMATOES, MOZZARELLA, FRESH BASIL, SERVED OVER A SMALL GREEN SALAD WITH OLIVE OIL BALSAMIC VINEGAR DRESSING

6
Roulade de Fromage de Chevre
WARM GOAT CHEESE SALAD WITH POTATO ROULADE, SERVED OVER A GREEN SALAD WITH FRENCH DRESSING

6
Salade de Chevre Frisse
LENTIL BEAN FRISEE SALAD WITH GOAT CHEESE WITH A DUSTED PEPPER RED WINE SHALLOT VINAIGRETTE

FRUITS DE MER

A tower of crustacean power, complete with clams, mussels, oysters, shrimp, and often crowned with a cooked lobster tail. It's a low-fat, high-protein treat that's as fun to eat as it is healthy, as long as you keep the bounty of the sea away from the ramekins of melted butter and flavored mayonnaise.

6
Pate de Foie Gras
FOIE PATE SERVED OVER A SMALL SALAD AND GARLIC TOAST POINTS

7
Escargots Au Beurre D'ail
ESCARGOTS SAUTEED WITH GARLIC, BUTTER, HERBES AND CHAMPAGNE

36
Fruits De Mer
ASSORTED SHELLFISH WITH A VARIETY OF DIPPING SAUCES

ENTREES

13
Truit
LEMON THYME
ROASTED WHOLE TROUT, SPINACH,
SHALLOTS, IN A CHAMPAGNE BEURRE
BLANC SAUCE

15
Saumon
PAN SEARED SALMON SERVED WITH
ASPARAGUS, CARROTS JULIENNE OF
VEGETABLES, IN BEURRE BLANC
SAUCE

10
Lotte
SAUTEED MONK FISH IN A BEURRE
BLANC SAUCE GREEN PEPPER SAUCE,
SERVED WITH VEGETABLES AND
MASHED POTATOES

15
Moules Provencales
STEAMED MUSSELS IN A WHITE WINE
GARLIC AND FRESH TOMATO SAUCE,
SERVED WITH FRENCH FRIES

VIANDES

15
Steak & Fries
GRILLED NEW YORK STRIP STEAK IN A
CLASSIC BEARNAISE SAUCE SERVED
WITH SMALL SALAD AND FRENCH FRIES

19
Filet Mignon
GRILLED FILET MIGNON, SERVED
WITH BABY VEGETABLES, SPINACH
AND MASHED POTATOES

25
Steak Tartare
FRESH CHOPPED BEEF FILET
SERVED WITH MIXED GREENS

21
Canard Mandarin Cerise
ROASTED LONG ISLAND DUCK,
SERVED WITH CORN POLENTA CAKE
AND SAUTEED GARLIC SPINACH, WITH
CHERRY COMPOTE SAUCE

16
Confit of Wild Boar Shoulder
WITH SPAËZLES, MUSHROOMS,
CHESTNUTS AND BLACK CURRANTS

12
Blanc de Poulet Grand-mere
ORGANIC ROASTED CHICKEN
BREAST, SERVED WITH JULIANNE OF
VEGETABLES AND MASHED POTATOES,
IN A TOMATO SAUCE

14
Linguini Aux Fruits de Mer
LINGUINI WITH SEA FOOD
(CUTTLEFISH, SQUID, OCTOPUS,
SHRIMP, SURINI AND MUSSELS),
FRESH TOMATOES, GARLIC AND BASIL

13
Pappardelle pappardelle,
WILD MUSHROOMS, SAGE BUTTER
SWEET PEAS, SHAVED PECORINO
ROMANO CHEESE

DESSERT

10 New York Cheese Cake
IN A BERRIES SAUCE

10 Crème Brulée

10 Chocolate Mousse
TOPPED WITH WHIPPED CREAM

STEAK TARTARE

Raw beef usually topped with raw egg.
If you can stomach the thought, go for it:
The huge protein goes a long way in
filling you up, and because it's made with a
lean cut of meat, it's relatively low in fat.

ROASTED

Meaning coated in olive oil,
salt, and pepper and cooked
in an oven. A standard bistro
cooking technique, order it
when it's applied to fish
or chicken, not duck or lamb.

CONFIT

"To cook slowly in
its own fat" is the
belt-loosening
translation here.

STEAK FRITES

A fatty cut of beef, either a rib eye or a
hanger steak, topped with a pad of flavored butter
or a butter-based bérnaise sauce and flanked
by a pile of fries. The damage: 1,200 calories and 70
grams of fat. Start with a steak tartare instead;
it should satisfy your red meat craving
for a quarter of the calories.

CRÈME BRULÉE

Egg yolks, heavy cream,
and sugar. Lighten the
load with an extra spoon,
or opt for a fruit-filled
crepe instead.

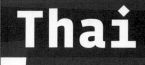

Thai

APPETIZERS

CRISPY SPRING ROLLS (Vegetables) $5.95   FRIED WONTON (Chicken) $6.95
STEAMED DUMPLING (Chicken or vegetables) $5.95   POTSTICKERS (Chicken or vegetables) $5.95
SHU MAI (Pork & shrimp) $5.95   MEEKROB (Chicken or tofu) $7.95
VIETNAMESE SPRING ROLLS (Shrimp or tofu) $6.95   FRIED SHRIMP ROLLS $6.95
CHICKEN SATE $7.95   PEKING DUCK ROLL $6.95

SALADS

HOUSE SALAD $6.95   CHINESE SALAD $8.95
THAI CHICKEN SALAD With chicken breast topped with peanut sauce $8.95
TOFU SALAD Steamed tofu tossed with spicy lime dressing $8.95
SPICY CHICKEN SALAD (LARB) Minced chicken tossed with spicy lime dressing $9.95
YUM WOON SEN Glass noodle with chicken tossed with spicy lime dressing $8.95
YUM YAI Boiled chicken, egg, and shrimp over a bed of lettuce topped with
fresh peanuts and sweet & sour sauce $9.95
SPICY BBQ BEEF SALAD Tossed with spicy lime dressing $9.95
GRILLED SHRIMP AND ASPARAGUS SALAD Tossed with house vinaigrette dressing $9.95
BBQ DUCK SALAD $9.95   SPICY DUCK SALAD Tossed with spicy lime dressing $9.95
SPICY SHRIMP SALAD Tossed with spicy lime dressing $9.95
SPICY SEAFOOD SALAD Shrimp, scallops, mussels, and crap with spicy lime dressing...$10.95

VEGETABLES & TOFU

SAUTEED SPINACH $10.95   SZECHWAN STRING BEANS $10.95
GARLIC EGGPLANT $10.95   ORANGE TOFU .$10.95
RED CURRY VEGETABLES $10.95   STEAMED VEGETABLE PLATE $10.95
VEGETABLE DELUXE Sauteed asparagus, snow peas, baby bok choy, and broccoli $10.95

SPECIALTIES

THAI BBQ CHICKEN .$10.95   BBQ PORK RIBS. $10.95
ORANGE CHICKEN $11.95   TERIYAKI CHICKEN $10.95
DAVID'S SPECIAL Spicy minced chicken and fried egg on the top of coconut rice $12.95
CRYSTAL'S SPECIAL Garlic pork over chicken fried rice .$12.95
PAULINA'S SPECIAL Ginger chicken and vegetables with steamed white & brown rice $12.95
PAUL'S SPECIAL Shrimp with garlic served with asparagus and noodles $14.95
RYAN'S SPECIAL Sauteed bok choy, broccoli, and chicken with steamed brown & wild rice $12.95
MARK'S SPECIAL Stir fried flat rice noodles with scallops and eggs $12.95
FRESH ASPARAGUS & CHICKEN $12.95   MONGOLIAN BBQ BEEF $12.95
HONEY DUCK Topped with house honey and hoisin sauce $12.95
GARLIC SCALLOPS $12.95   FISH WITH BLACK BEAN SAUCE $12.95
THAI CHILLI FISH Lightly fried and topped with thai chilli sauce... $12.95
FILET OF SOLE Lightly fried and topped with house curry sauce $12.95
STEAMED FILLET OF SOLE With house ginger and steamed vegetables $12.95
PLA LARD PRIK Crispy snapper with chili, garlic and tamarind $12.95

ROLLS (SPRING AND SUMMER)

Spring = deep-fried.
Summer = not deep-fried.
Now choose accordingly.

SATAY

Lean grilled meat on a stick slathered in a spicy peanut sauce. Seriously satisfying, low-fat food.

TOFU

Tofu acts like a soybean sponge, sucking up anything it comes into contact with. When it's fried, like it is here, that translates into a heavy dose of oil and little else. Ask for it sauteed, or stick to vegetables.

VEGETABLES

Laced with ginger, garlic, and chilies, Thai-style vegetables pack huge flavor for few calories. Try splitting an entrée with a companion and sharing a side of sizzling vegetables to round out the meal.

PLA LARD PRIK

The crispy whole snapper's "crispy" part comes from its bath in a wok of hot, bubbling oil. Eat the whole thing with rice and the meal tops out around 900 calories.

ENTRÉE

CHOICE OF CHICKEN, BEEF, TOFU, OR VEGETABLES $10.95   CHOICE OF SHRIMP $12.95

GARLIC & BLACK PEPPER Served with steamed vegetables

SPICY BASIL Served with steamed vegetables

KUNG PAO Roasted peanuts, scallion, and blacken chilli pepper

CASHEW NUT Roasted cashew nuts sautéed with scallion

BROCCOLI Sauteed with a touch of garlic

SWEET & SOUR Pineapple, union, carrot, and bell pepper in special pungent sa

BLACK BEAN SAUCE Our most famous sauce, bell pepper, and white onion

YELLOW CURRY (KANG KAREE) With potato, carrot, and onion

RED CURRY (PANANG) Spicy house curry sauce

GREEN CURRY Our popular curry dish from Bangkok

MIXED VEGETABLES Sauteed with a touch of garlic

PRIK KING Green beans in spicy red sauce

GREEN CURRY

Thai curries, regardless of color, are based around coconut milk. While high in saturated fat, most of that comes from lauric acid, which has been shown in more than 60 studies to decrease your risk of cardiovascular disease. Pick a lean protein like shrimp or chicken, and this makes for a healthier option than many of the noodle-based dishes.

RICE

THAI FRIED RICE   SPICY BASIL FRIED RICE

CHOICE OF CHICKEN, BEEF, TOFU, OR VEGETABLES $8.95   CHOICE OF SHRIMP $10.95

SPECIAL BROWN RICE Stir fried brown & wild rice with vegetables, and eggs $10.95

SEAFOOD FRIED RICE (shrimp, scallops, crab) $12.95

FRIED RICE

Nearly as oil-soaked as its Chinese counterpart.

THE NOODLE STATION

PAD THAI Our most popular noodle dish

SPICY BASIL NOODLE Flat rice noodle with bell pepper and onion

RAD NA Flat rice noodle topped with house gravy sauce

LO MEIN Stir fried noodle with vegetables

CHOICE OF CHICKEN, BEEF, TOFU, OR VEGETABLES $9.95

CRISPY NOODLE WITH CHICKEN & VEGETABLES Topped with house ginger sauce $12.95

CRISPY NOODLE WITH SEAFOOD & VEGETABLES Topped with house ginger sauce..$14.95

PAD THAI

An average portion of this popular noodle entrée can be 600 calories, but it's usually very low in saturated fat, making it a pretty good option.

BEVERAGES

THAI ICED TEA

With non- dairy creamer $2.95

THAI ICED COFFEE

With non- dairy creamer $2.95

REGULAR ICED TEA $2.95

LEMONADE $2.95

ORANGE JUICE $3.95

CRANBERRY JUICE $2.95

SODAS (COKE, SPRITE, DIET COKE) $2.95

SPARKLING WATER $3.00

BOTTLE WATER $5.00

BEERS

DOMESTIC BEER $3.25

IMPORTED BEER $3.75

HOT SAKE $3.75   HOT TEA $9.50

WINES

GLASS $5.95

BOTTLE .$22.00

WHITE WINE CHARDONNAY, SAUVIGNON BLANC, PINOT GRIGIO

RED WINE MERLOT, CARBERNET

PLUM WINE

THAI ICED TEA

Any potential benefits of the brute-strength black tea are hopelessly diluted by the addition of sweetened condensed milk and a few fistfuls of sugar. Sip this and your blood sugar levels will soar, which signals your body to start storing fat.

Salad Bar

Build a Better Salad

If you're on the run from unnecessary calories, you might think you'll find safe haven at the salad bar. But beware: Modern food manufacturers have found a way to screw up even this sure thing. Sliced meats, croutons (white bread fried in oil), and other nutritional imposters abound.

But a really great salad can be the best nutritional punch of all. Here, we've outlined the absolute healthiest salad you can make: although it's slightly high in calories (at 570), it packs megadoses of vitamins A and C, heart-healthy fats, and 42 grams of muscle-building protein—that's as much as in a New York strip steak. Here's the breakdown:

CRUNCH
Croutons lend texture but do nothing for your body except bloat it. Opt for thinly sliced red or yellow bell peppers: more vitamin C, and a deep crunch.

LETTUCE
You need something hearty enough to hold the weight of your salad. Mixed greens bruise easily. So try romaine—a nutritional powerhouse, with a ton of fiber and vitamins A and C. Tear or chop it into pieces.

BONUS PRODUCE
Start with a cup of steamed green beans. Add to that 1/2 cup of chopped tomatoes for your lycopene fix. A handful of olives brings a hit of heart-healthy monounsaturated fats.

EGGS-TRA PROTEIN
Hard-boiled eggs provide a protein boost. For a bright, creamy yolk, cook an egg in gently simmering water for 8 minutes. Want more protein and fiber? Add 1/2 cup of canned chickpeas to the salad.

VESSEL
Yes, even the serving dish matters. A Cornell University study found that a salad heaped on a plate creates the perception of a more substantial meal than one hidden deep in a bowl.

PROTEIN
Wild Planet (1wildplanet.com) offers wild albacore tuna with a big dose of protein, heart-helping omega-3 fats, and $1/3$ of the mercury found in most canned stuff. Or sub in grilled chicken breast.

DRESSING
If you're at home, make this healthy vinaigrette: In a jar, combine $1/3$ cup olive oil with $1/4$ cup red wine vinegar, 2 Tbsp. minced onion, 1 Tbsp. Dijon mustard, and a bit of cracked black pepper. Screw on the top and shake.

Dress Properly

You know olive oil is good for you. But how does it stack up against other oils as a salad dressing, or even for cooking? One way to judge an oil is by its ratio of monounsaturated fat to saturated fat: The higher, the better, says the American Dietetic Association. So before you fire up the stove, check out these winners.

CANOLA OIL (10:1)
It has the lowest amount of saturated fat among common cooking oils but fewer heart-healthy monounsaturated fats. Canola is the top choice for sautéing or frying because it doesn't smoke at high temperatures and has a neutral taste. To fuel fat loss, try Enova® oil. It's a special combination of canola and soybean oils that your body will be more likely to burn for energy than store as fat.

OLIVE OIL (5:1)
It contains antioxidants and monounsaturated fats that help keep your cholesterol low and your arteries clear. Unfortunately, olive oil has a relatively low smoke temperature, meaning it's not great for frying or high-temperature cooking.

PEANUT OIL (5:2) Peanut oil isn't overly high in saturated fat, and its great taste and elevated smoke temperature make it an excellent choice for cooking.

CORN OIL (2:1) Versatile-but-bland corn oil is low in saturated fat but places fourth for overall health.

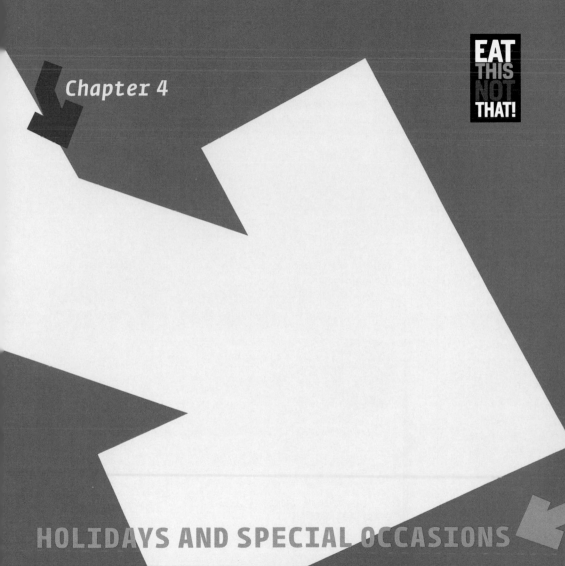

EAT
THIS
NOT
THAT!

Chapter 4

HOLIDAYS AND SPECIAL OCCASIONS

Thanksgiving

Burn off the Bird

More food is consumed in the United States on Thanksgiving Day than on any other day of the year. Skip the gym and work off the feast with the family. Here's how:

TURKEY AND GRAVY:
● 55 minutes of touch football

MASHED POTATOES AND GRAVY:
● 4.5-mile-walk with the family

PUMPKIN PIE WITH WHIPPED CREAM:
● 35 minutes of raking at your parents' place

STUFFING:
● 40 minutes of playing with the kids

DINNER ROLL:
● 30 minutes of dish washing

CRANBERRY SAUCE:
● 50 minutes of movie watching

Eat This

Turkey Breast Dinner, 6 oz

731 calories
61 g protein
85 g carbohydrates
20 g fat
(11 g saturated)
1,240 sodium

1 medium slice pumpkin pie
with low-fat whipped cream
335 calories
15 g fat
(6.5 g saturated)
42 g carbohydrates

⅔ cup mashed potatoes
⅓ cup turkey gravy
1 dinner roll
1 cup green bean casserole
¼ cup homemade cranberry sauce

Not That!

Dark Meat Turkey Dinner, 6 oz

1,279 calories
62 g protein
159 g carbohydrates
48 g fat
(22 g saturated)
1,890 sodium

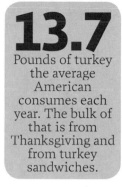

13.7
Pounds of turkey the average American consumes each year. The bulk of that is from Thanksgiving and from turkey sandwiches.

LEFTOVERS

1 serving turkey breast

on whole grain bread with lettuce and cranberry sauce and ½ cup green bean casserole

530 calories
20 g fat
(7 g saturated)
1,015 mg sodium

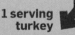

1 serving turkey

on Kaiser roll with mayo, ⅔ cup mashed potatoes, and ⅓ cup turkey gravy

665 calories
30 g fat
(7 g saturated)
1,300 mg sodium

1 cup stuffing
⅔ cup sweet potatoes with marshmallow topping
½ cup corn
1 slice jellied cranberry sauce

1 small slice pecan pie
375 calories
28 g fat
(6 g saturated)
55 g carbohydrates

Pie Chart

Nothing's more American than Mom and apple pie. But food manufacturers would rather have us noshing on Twinkies® and Ding Dongs® than old-fashioned pies. That's bad, because Mom's pies are made with real fruit, which packs massive doses of vitamins, minerals, and fiber, while Twinkies pack massive doses of something called polysorbate 60, a petroleum product used to construct plastic bottles. Yikes. If you're going to indulge, go home-style and whip up one of these natural wonders instead. (Use real butter instead of margarine or Crisco® for the

BLUEBERRY PIE
473 calories, 19 g fat.

Blueberries carry a rich lode of antioxidants, those all-purpose compounds that help your body fight heart disease and cancer; the berries' flavonoids may help your eyesight, balance, coordination, and short-term memory.

PUMPKIN PIE
465 calories, 25 g fat.

Pumpkin is loaded with carotenoids, which help prevent heart disease and cancer. That slice is a big dose of beta carotene, which may help fight prostate cancer, protect your eyesight, and keep mucous membranes resistant to infection.

APPLE PIE
525 calories, 19 g fat.

Phytonutrients in apples may help fight colon and liver cancers. The flavonoid quercetin can reduce your risk of lung and prostate cancers, and it strengthens your immune cells.

LEMON MERINGUE PIE

562 calories, 20 g fat.

You'll get half an egg per slice, and eggs have choline, a nutrient that's been shown to improve memory. The antioxidants in lemons ward off aging and infection. And that vitamin C means no scurvy for you!

CHERRY PIE

507 calories, 19 g fat.

Cherries are chock-full of anthocyanins, which increase the strength of blood vessels and may relieve muscle pain and slow the development of arthritis and gout. They may even protect your lungs from smoke.

PECAN PIE

678 calories, 51 g fat.

A big, goopy dilemma. Loads of fat, but almost 90 percent of the fat in these nuts is unsaturated, and pecans can reduce your levels of bad cholesterol (LDL) and raise your good cholesterol (HDL).

crust, to cut down on trans fats.) These stats are for a mom-size wedge, one-sixth of a 9-inch pie. Or two slivers, which we've seen you eat.

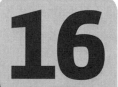

16

Grams of fat saved by baking a pie using Keebler® Graham Ready Crust instead of Pillsbury® Refrigerated Pie Crust.

For more great food swaps, nutritional secrets, quick and simple recipes, weight-loss tactics, and the latest breaking news on staying lean and feeling great, go to *menshealth.com/eatthis*

Christmas Dinner

Eat This

Beef Tenderloin Dinner, 8 oz

950 calories
38 g fat
(17 g saturated)
900 mg sodium

Make your fondue with dark chocolate rather than milk—you'll get more antioxidants and less sugar out of dessert.

Roasted trumps mashed every time in the potato department. Tossed simply with olive oil, salt, and pepper, they'll save you 100 calories over the mashed.

Horseradish sauce

Roasted new potatoes

Green beans with almonds

Dinner roll with butter

Chocolate fondue with fresh fruit

Glass of red wine

Not That!

Honey-Baked Ham Dinner, 8 oz

1,565 calories
90 g fat
(45 g saturated)
2,500 mg sodium

Cornbread is loaded with sugar, which pushes its calorie count past a common dinner roll.

Mashed potates with gravy

Salad with croutons and vinaigrette

Cornbread with butter

Slice of cheesecake

Glass of beer

Ham is fattier than beef tenderloin to begin with, but the candy-like glaze tacks on a heap of added sugars.

New Year's Eve

Eat This

12 large shrimp

with 2 tablespoons cocktail sauce

165 calories
<1 g fat
(0 g saturated)
480 mg sodium

A recent Spanish study found that a glass of sparkling wine can help reduce heart-threatening inflammation.

Shrimp are essentially fat-free and protein-packed, which makes them one of the few foods you can gorge on without paying the price. But limit yourself on the cocktail sauce—it's mostly tomatoes, but it's heavy on sodium.

Other Picks

8 melon balls wrapped in prosciutto

220 calories
11 g fat (4 g saturated)
900 mg sodium

Glass of champagne, 6 oz

130 calories
0 g fat
6 g carbohydrates

Not That!

Crab cake

290 calories
19 g fat
(4 g saturated)
600 mg sodium

An 8 oz splash
of tonic water has
nearly as much sugar as
some regular soft
drinks. Opt for diet,
if available:
it's sugar-free.

The crab lumps
are bound in mayo,
then rolled in breadcrumbs
and fried, which is
why only one of these does
more damage than a
dozen lean shrimp.

Other Passes

383 calories
15 g fat (6 g saturated)
1,400 mg sodium

1 potato pancake with smoked salmon, sour cream, and caviar

240 calories
0 g fat
16 g carbohydrates

Gin and tonic, 8 oz

177

Halloween

Eat This

Skittles® (fun size)
80 calories
1 g fat (1 g saturated)
15 g sugars

These rainbow-colored candies aren't perfect, but they have a fraction of the sugar and fat found in Starburst®.

Tootsie® Caramel Apple Pop
60 calories
.5 g fat (0 g saturated)
11 g sugars

PayDay® (fun size)
90 calories
5 g fat (.5 g saturated)
10 g sugars

PayDay® has the lowest level of saturated fat in the candy bar aisle.

Whoppers® (6 pieces)
60 calories
2.5 g fat (2 g saturated)
8 g sugars

Crunchy chocolate flavor with less sugar than Tootsie Rolls®.

3 Musketeers® bar
(fun size)
70 calories
2 g fat (1.5 g saturated)
11 g sugars

Twizzlers® Cherry Nibs
(22 pieces)
110 calories
0 g fat   18 g sugars

Less of a sugary assault on your system than candy corn, if eaten in moderation.

Not That!

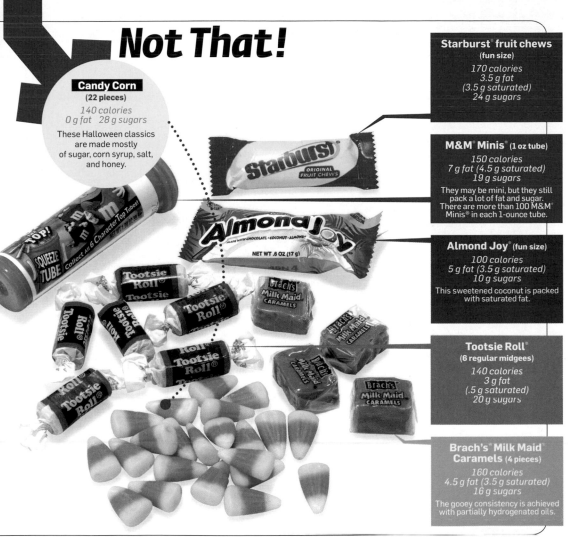

Candy Corn
(22 pieces)

140 calories
0 g fat   28 g sugars

These Halloween classics
are made mostly
of sugar, corn syrup, salt,
and honey.

Starburst® fruit chews
(fun size)

170 calories
3.5 g fat
(3.5 g saturated)
24 g sugars

M&M® Minis® (1 oz tube)

150 calories
7 g fat (4.5 g saturated)
19 g sugars

They may be mini, but they still
pack a lot of fat and sugar.
There are more than 100 M&M®
Minis® in each 1-ounce tube.

Almond Joy® (fun size)

100 calories
5 g fat (3.5 g saturated)
10 g sugars

This sweetened coconut is packed
with saturated fat.

Tootsie Roll®
(6 regular midgees)

140 calories
3 g fat
(.5 g saturated)
20 g sugars

Brach's™ Milk Maid®
Caramels (4 pieces)

160 calories
4.5 g fat (3.5 g saturated)
16 g sugars

The gooey consistency is achieved
with partially hydrogenated oils.

Your Easter Basket

Eat This

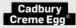

Cadbury Creme Egg®

150 calories
5 g fat (3 g saturated)
22 g sugars

The Classic Cadbury egg beats the newer chocolate version by 30 calories and 3 grams of fat.

THE ORIGINAL GOURMET JELLY BEAN®
20 FLAVORS

Jordan almonds (12 pieces)	Milky Way® Midnight™ bar	Gummi Bears (14 pieces)	Hershey's® Cookies 'n' Crème™ bar	Jelly Belly® Jelly Beans (14 pieces)	Hershey's Hugs® (9 pieces)
200 calories	*220 calories*	*140 calories*	*80 calories*	*150 calories*	*210 calories*
7 g fat	*8 g fat*	*0 g fat*	*4.5 g fat*	*0 g fat*	*12 g fat*
(1 g saturated)	*(5 g saturated)*		*(2.5 g saturated)*		*(7 g saturated)*
26 g sugars	*29 g sugars*	*22 g sugars*	*9 g sugars*	*27 g sugars*	*21 g sugars*

Not That!

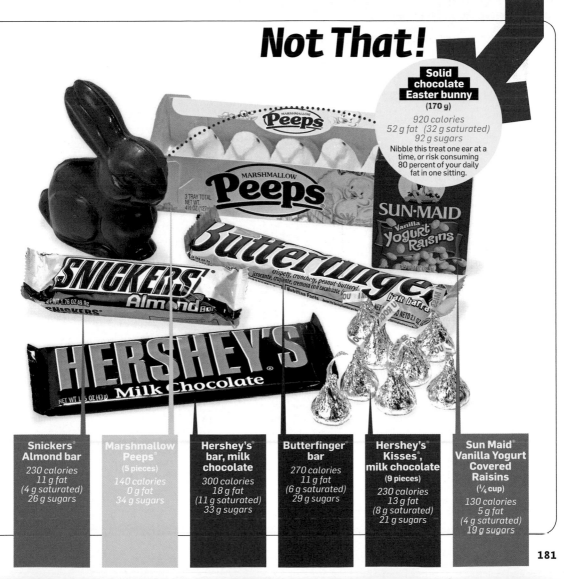

Solid chocolate Easter bunny
(170 g)

920 calories
52 g fat (32 g saturated)
92 g sugars

Nibble this treat one ear at a time, or risk consuming 80 percent of your daily fat in one sitting.

Snickers® Almond bar

230 calories
11 g fat
(4 g saturated)
26 g sugars

Marshmallow Peeps®
(5 pieces)

140 calories
0 g fat
34 g sugars

Hershey's® bar, milk chocolate

300 calories
18 g fat
(11 g saturated)
33 g sugars

Butterfinger® bar

270 calories
11 g fat
(6 g saturated)
29 g sugars

Hershey's® Kisses®, milk chocolate
(9 pieces)

230 calories
13 g fat
(8 g saturated)
21 g sugars

Sun Maid® Vanilla Yogurt Covered Raisins
(¼ cup)

130 calories
5 g fat
(4 g saturated)
19 g sugars

181

Valentine's Day
Eat This

Fannie May® Marshmallow
fluff and dark chocolate (1 piece)

78 calories
2.5 g fat (1.5 g saturated)
11 g sugars

Although high in sugar, airy marshmallow delivers fewer calories and fat grams than fudge fillings.

Vanilla caramel
(1 piece)

70 calories
3 g fat
(2 g saturated)
10 g sugars

Less than half the calories and sugar of a tall caramel macchiato. Caramel is made by boiling milk, sugar, butter, oil, syrup, vanilla, and glucose gum.

Chocolate-covered cherry
(1 piece)

60 calories
2 g fat
(1.5 g saturated)
8 g sugars

Cherries are chock-full of anthocyanins, which increase the strength of blood vessels and may relieve muscle pain.

Lemon cream
(1 piece)

65 calories
2 g fat
(1 g saturated)
10 g sugars

A combination of sweetness and tartness without the drippy, sugary syrup of other chocolate-covered fruits.

Milk chocolate mint meltaway
(1 piece)

48 calories
1.5 g fat
(1 g saturated)
7.5 g sugars

Creamy peppermint flavor with less fat than a scoop of mint chocolate chip ice cream or a Mint Milano® cookie.

Chocolate-covered citrus peel (1 piece)

43 calories
1.5 g fat
(1 g saturated)
4.5 g sugars

90 percent of citrus-peel oils consist of d-limonene, an antioxidant that's been shown to kill cancer cells.

Not That!

Fannie May® Chocolate fudge
(1 piece)

120 calories
5 g fat (3 g saturated)
17 g sugars

Fudge is a chocolate brick made almost entirely of butter and sugar.

LITTLE TRICK

When you present her with that box of chocolates, save a few for yourself. A Johns Hopkins study found that the nitric oxide–boosting compounds found in chocolate can help trigger and maintain erections.

French nougat
(1 piece)

125 calories
5 g fat
(2 g saturated)
14 g sugars

Nougat is mostly honey, cut with roasted nuts, adding to the high sugar count here.

Chocolate toffee
(1 piece)

80 calories
6 g fat
(3.5 g saturated)
6.5 g sugars

Toffee is made by boiling molasses with butter and milk, then letting it harden until crisp. Most toffee candies will be high in saturated fat.

Peanut butter smooth truffle

55 calories
6 g fat
(4 g saturated)
8 g sugars

Avoid peanut butter truffles, which are high in sugar and fat and low in heart-healthy monounsaturated fat found naturally in peanuts.

Cappuccino truffle
(1 piece)

140 calories
8 g fat
(7 g saturated)
15 g sugars

This rich truffle has double the fat and sugar of a real cappuccino, delivering coffee flavor without the antioxidants.

The Fourth of July

Eat This

Filet mignon, 6 oz

260 calories
11 g fat
(4 g saturated)
200 mg sodium

It doesn't get any leaner in the beef world than tenderloin. Even if you nixed the cheese and wrapped the burger in lettuce, it would still lose the battle of the barbie.

Coleslaw (4 oz)

150 calories
8 g fat (1 g saturated)
350 mg sodium

Both coleslaw and potato salad are vehicles for the same fatty passenger, mayo. So it all comes down to which one makes for a healthier vehicle. Cabbage is dense with sulforaphane, a chemical that boosts your body's production of enzymes that fend off cancer.

Tortilla chips and guacamole
(about 12 chips)

140 calories
9 g fat (3 g saturated)
460 mg sodium

Ranch and guac might have nearly the same amount of overall fat, but avocados are packed with heart-healthy monounsaturated fats— ranch dressing is not.

Baked beans
(¾ cup, made without bacon)

150 calories
1.5 g fat (0 g saturated)
350 mg sodium

Sure, the beans have a few more calories, but they're significantly lower in fat and pack huge protein and fiber to keep you feeling fuller longer. Plus, studies have found that red beans are among the most antioxidant-dense foods.

Watermelon
(1 medium-sized hunk)

46 calories
10 g sugars

Watermelon is loaded with potassium and lycopene, which has been shown to help fight off both breast cancer and prostate cancer.

Not That!
Cheeseburger, 4 oz

630 calories
41 g fat
(15 g saturated)
735 mg sodium

Drop the cheese and form your patties with 95% lean beef and you'll cut 250 calories and 25 grams of fat from the meal.

Peach (1 whole)

68 calories
15 g sugars

It's not that peaches are bad—even though 15 grams of sugar is more than most fruit has—it's just that watermelon, cantaloupe, and blueberries all offer more nutritional bang for the bite.

Corn on the cob
with ½ tablespoon of butter

180 calories
10 grams fat
(5 grams saturated)
150 mg sodium

The corn itself isn't a high-impact food, but it offers little for you nutritionally, and its best friend is butter. Two good reasons to reach for the beans instead.

Veggies
and ranch dip

160 calories
10 g fat (6 g saturated)
370 mg sodium

Who are you fooling? Everyone knows those carrot sticks are just there to bring the ranch from bowl to mouth.

Potato salad
(4 oz)

180 calories
12 g fat
(2 g saturated)
430 mg sodium

Potatoes and mayo pack a one-two punch of carbs and fat. For a lighter option, go with a German-style mustard-based potato salad.

185

The Ballpark
Eat This

Hot dog
with relish, ketchup, and mustard
280 calories
15 g fat (5 g saturated)
1,250 mg sodium

Moderate amounts of beer can help to raise HDL (good) cholesterol and lower insulin resistance. Moderate amounts of soft drinks will raise belly fat and lower energy levels.

Assuming you can limit yourself to one, and you skip the chili and cheese, hot dogs are one of the best ballpark entrée options.

Neapolitan ice cream sandwich
190 calories
7 g fat (3.5 g saturated)
15 g sugars

Cracker Jack® (1 box)
420 calories
7 g fat (0 g saturated)
240 g sodium

Regular beer (12 oz)
139 calories
0 g fat
12 g carbohydrates

186

Not That!

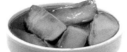

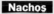

Nachos
692 calories
38 g fat (16 g saturated)
1,632 mg sodium

Malts and soft serve come in huge portion sizes, which makes a relatively small ice cream sandwich the best choice here.

Want to have your nachos and eat them too? Ask for the cheese sauce on the side and dip sparingly.

Large soft pretzel
with cheese dip
570 calories
11.5 g fat (3 g saturated)
2,340 mg sodium

Cola (16 oz)
155 calories
0 g fat
49 g carbohydrates

French vanilla soft serve ice cream (1 cup)
380 calories
22 g fat (13 g saturated)
36 g sugars

Black Friday at the Mall

Eat This

Auntie Anne's™ Cinnamon Sugar Pretzel

without butter

350 calories
2 g fat (0 g saturated)
16 g sugars

McDonald's® Fruit 'n Yogurt Parfait

160 calories
2 g fat
(1 g saturated)
21 g sugars

TCBY® Non-Fat Frozen Yogurt

(small)

110 calories
0 g fat
20 g sugars

Panda Express® Mushroom Chicken with Mixed Vegetables

200 calories
10 g fat
(2 g saturated)
690 mg sodium

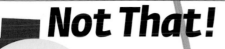

Not That!

Cinnabon® Classic Cinnamon Roll

730 calories
24 g fat (8 g saturated,
5 g trans fat)
49 g sugar

Sbarro New York Style Thin Crust Chicken and Vegetable Pizza
(1 slice)

530 calories
17 g fat
1,260 mg sodium

Orange Julius®
(16 oz)

220 calories
1 g fat
(0g saturated)
50 g sugars

Mrs. Fields® Semi-Sweet Chocolate Chip Cookie

210 calories
10 g fat
(5 g saturated)
18 g sugars

189

The Movies

Eat This

Raisinets (1.6 oz bag)

190 calories
8 g fat (5 g saturated)
26 g sugars

Raisinets deliver 1 gram of fiber—mix half the box with a handful of natural raisins to add 2 more.

Junior Mints
(one box, 40 grams)

170 calories
3 g fat (2.5 g saturated)
32 g sugars

Tootsie Roll Industries now also makes Junior Caramels, a blend of milk chocolate and soft caramel.

Buncha Crunch (⅓ cup)

180 calories
8 g fat (5 g saturated)
20 g sugars

Munching a serving of Buncha Crunch instead of devouring an original Crunch bar will save you 4 grams of fat.

Good & Plenty (1.5 oz)

150 calories
0 g fat   23 g sugars

Save this treat for R-rated films: Chicago researchers found that the aroma of black licorice increases bloodflow to the nether regions.

Swedish Fish (1.5 oz box)

140 calories
0 g fat   28 g sugars

In the vast category of candy made of mostly sugar and corn syrup, these fish are fat-free and contain less sugar than Skittles or Twizzlers.

Popcorn
(10-cup serving)

550 calories
31 g fat (5 g saturated)
972 mg sodium

The buttery topping adds 180 calories to a small and 350 to a large, so go easy on the "golden flavor."

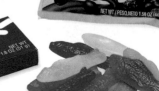

Creamy mints in pure chocolate

Junior Mints

Net Wt 4.75 oz (134 g)

On the Go!
Nestlé Buncha CRUNCH!

Nestlé RAISINETS
Nestlé Milk Chocolate ★ California Raisins

Good & Plenty

Not That!

Nachos
(6 to 8 nacho chips
with cheese)

608 calories
34 g fat (14 g saturated)
1,736 mg sodium

The orange goo is molten
trans fat masquerading
as cheese.

Chocolate Pretzel Flipz
(2 oz bag)

260 calories
10 g fat (6 g saturated)
20 g sugars

The White Fudge Flipz are even
worse, adding 3 grams of saturated
fat and 6 grams of sugar.

M&Ms
(1 bag, 48 grams)

240 calories
10 g fat (6 g saturated)
31 g sugars

The same amount
of sugar as the Junior Mints,
but double the fat.

Dots
(24 pieces)

280 calories
0 g fat   42 g sugars

They cram nearly 2 grams of sugar
into every Dot.

Cherry Twizzlers
(8 twists)

320 calories
2 g fat (0 g saturated)
42 g sugars

You're better off buying Twizzlers
Cherry Nibs®. A package of Nibs
has 100 fewer calories.

Reese's Pieces
(1.6 oz pack)

220 calories
11 g fat (8 g saturated)
23 g sugars

The "peanut butter" is actually a
peanut-flavored filling of sugar
and vegetable oil.

The Vending Machine

Eat This

Traditional Chex® Mix
(⅔ cup)

130 calories
4 g fat (.5 g saturated)
380 mg sodium

60 percent less fat than potato chips with a bit of fiber from the whole wheat cereal.

**Welch's®
Fruit Snacks,
Mixed Fruit**
(40 g)

130 calories
0 g fat
23 g sugars

They're made mostly of corn syrup, but these still contain 100% of your daily recommended vitamin C intake.

**Goldfish®
pretzels**
(1 oz bag)

100 calories
1 g fat
(0 g saturated)
410 mg sodium

More sodium, but less fat than the cheesy originals.

**York®
Peppermint
Pattie (1 patty)**

140 calories
2.5 g fat
(1.5 g saturated)
25 g sugars

**Ritz®
Peanut Butter
crackers**

190 calories
9 g fat
(1.5 g saturated)
370 mg sodium

All else being equal, peanut butter beats processed cheese every time.

**Rice Krispies
Treat**

90 calories
2.5 g fat
(1 g saturated)
8 g sugars

**Sun Chips®
French Onion**
(15 chips)

140 calories
6 g fat
(1 g saturated)
130 mg sodium

Twice the fiber of potato chips and 40 percent less fat.

Not That!

Combos® Cheddar Cheese crackers
(⅔ cup)

280 calories
12 g fat (6 g saturated)
580 mg sodium

High in saturated fat and sodium. Opt for Cheez-Its® to cut back on both.

Kit Kat Crisp Wafers

Goldfish BAKED SNACK CRACKERS
Cheddar
NET WT 1.5 OZ (43g)

Reese's MILK CHOCOLATE 2 PEANUT BUTTER CUPS
NET WT 2.17 OZ 61.5g

Skittles

Ritz® Cheese crackers

200 calories
12 g fat
(2.5 g saturated)
460 mg sodium

Reese's® Peanut Butter Cups®
(2 cups)

280 calories
15 g fat
(6 g saturated)
26 g sugars

Funyuns®
(13 pieces)

140 calories
7 g fat
(1 g saturated)
240 mg sodium

All the odorous breath of onion flavoring, with none of the health benefits of real onions.

Tropical Skittles®
(2 oz bag)

250 calories
2.5 g fat
(2.5 g saturated)
47 g sugars

Kit Kat® bar

210 calories
11 g fat
(7 g saturated)
22 g sugars

Goldfish® crackers
(1 oz bag)

140 calories
6 g fat
(1.5 g saturated)
240 mg sodium

The flavor of cheese without any of the protein or calcium.

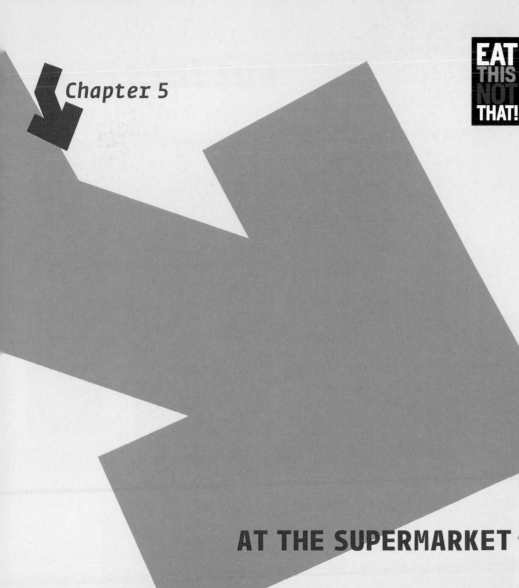

Chapter 5

EAT
THIS
NOT
THAT!

AT THE SUPERMARKET

Cereals

Eat This

When choosing cereals, the main goal is to maximize good nutrients like fiber and protein and minimize the junk like added sugars and high-fructose corn syrup. Make sure the stuff you start your day with has *at least* 3 grams of fiber (hopefully more!) and less than 10 grams of sugar per 1 cup serving.

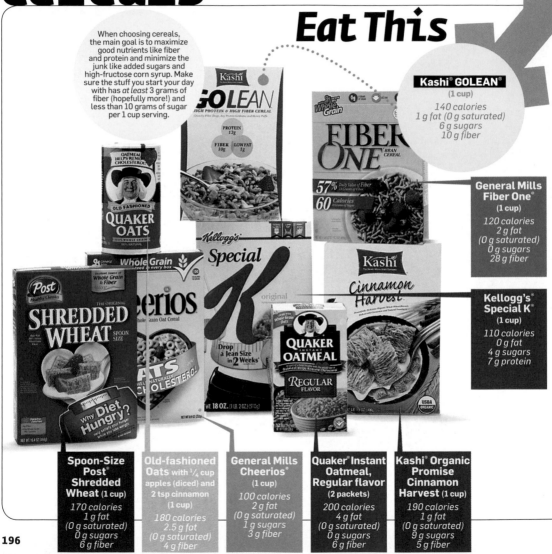

Kashi® GOLEAN®
(1 cup)

140 calories
1 g fat (0 g saturated)
6 g sugars
10 g fiber

General Mills Fiber One®
(1 cup)

120 calories
2 g fat
(0 g saturated)
0 g sugars
28 g fiber

Kellogg's® Special K®
(1 cup)

110 calories
0 g fat
4 g sugars
7 g protein

Spoon-Size Post® Shredded Wheat (1 cup)

170 calories
1 g fat
(0 g saturated)
0 g sugars
6 g fiber

Old-fashioned Oats with ¼ cup apples (diced) and 2 tsp cinnamon
(1 cup)

180 calories
2.5 g fat
(0 g saturated)
4 g fiber

General Mills Cheerios®
(1 cup)

100 calories
2 g fat
(0 g saturated)
1 g sugars
3 g fiber

Quaker® Instant Oatmeal, Regular flavor
(2 packets)

200 calories
4 g fat
(0 g saturated)
0 g sugars
6 g fiber

Kashi® Organic Promise Cinnamon Harvest (1 cup)

190 calories
1 g fat
(0 g saturated)
9 g sugars
5 g fiber

Not That!

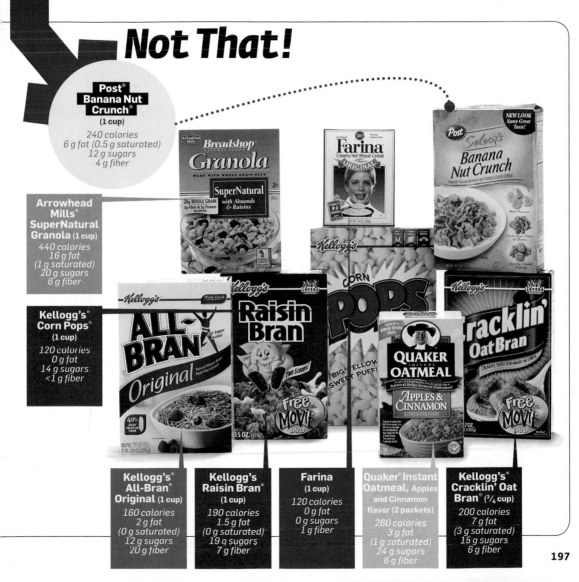

Post® Banana Nut Crunch® (1 cup)
240 calories
6 g fat (0.5 g saturated)
12 g sugars
4 g fiber

Arrowhead Mills® SuperNatural Granola (1 cup)
440 calories
16 g fat (1 g saturated)
20 g sugars
6 g fiber

Kellogg's® Corn Pops® (1 cup)
120 calories
0 g fat
14 g sugars
<1 g fiber

Kellogg's® All-Bran® Original (1 cup)
160 calories
2 g fat (0 g saturated)
12 g sugars
20 g fiber

Kellogg's Raisin Bran® (1 cup)
190 calories
1.5 g fat (0 g saturated)
19 g sugars
7 g fiber

Farina (1 cup)
120 calories
0 g fat
0 g sugars
1 g fiber

Quaker® Instant Oatmeal, Apples and Cinnamon flavor (2 packets)
260 calories
3 g fat (1 g saturated)
24 g sugars
6 g fiber

Kellogg's® Cracklin' Oat Bran® (³/₄ cup)
200 calories
7 g fat (3 g saturated)
15 g sugars
6 g fiber

197

Yogurt

Eat This

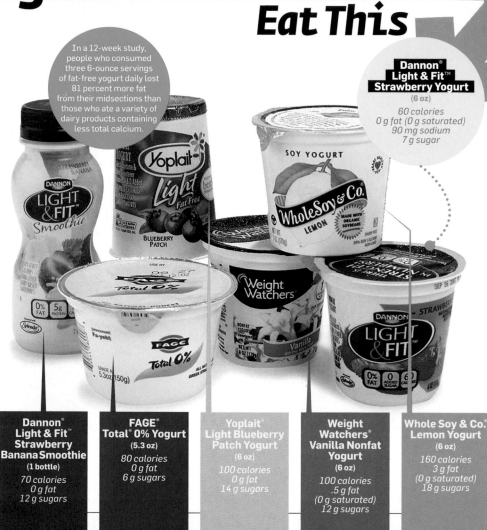

In a 12-week study, people who consumed three 6-ounce servings of fat-free yogurt daily lost 81 percent more fat from their midsections than those who ate a variety of dairy products containing less total calcium.

**Dannon®
Light & Fit™
Strawberry Yogurt**
(6 oz)

*60 calories
0 g fat (0 g saturated)
90 mg sodium
7 g sugar*

**Dannon®
Light & Fit™
Strawberry
Banana Smoothie**
(1 bottle)

*70 calories
0 g fat
12 g sugars*

**FAGE®
Total® 0% Yogurt**
(5.3 oz)

*80 calories
0 g fat
6 g sugars*

**Yoplait®
Light Blueberry
Patch Yogurt**
(6 oz)

*100 calories
0 g fat
14 g sugars*

**Weight
Watchers®
Vanilla Nonfat
Yogurt**
(6 oz)

*100 calories
.5 g fat
(0 g saturated)
12 g sugars*

**Whole Soy & Co.®
Lemon Yogurt**
(6 oz)

*160 calories
3 g fat
(0 g saturated)
18 g sugars*

Not That!

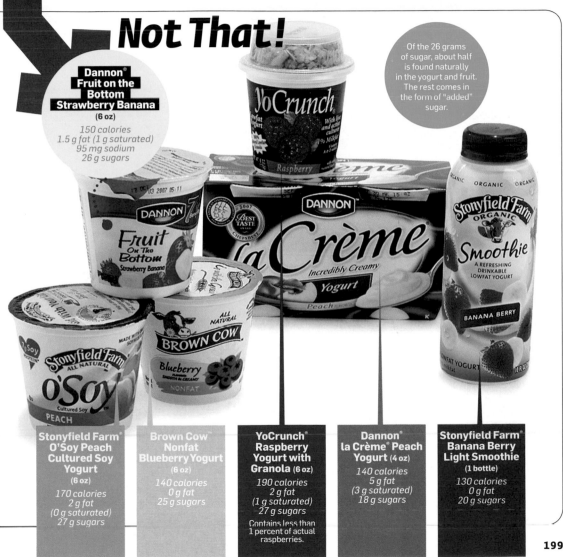

Of the 26 grams of sugar, about half is found naturally in the yogurt and fruit. The rest comes in the form of "added" sugar.

Dannon® Fruit on the Bottom Strawberry Banana
(6 oz)

150 calories
1.5 g fat (1 g saturated)
95 mg sodium
26 g sugars

Stonyfield Farm® O'Soy Peach Cultured Soy Yogurt
(6 oz)

170 calories
2 g fat
(0 g saturated)
27 g sugars

Brown Cow™ Nonfat Blueberry Yogurt
(6 oz)

140 calories
0 g fat
25 g sugars

YoCrunch® Raspberry Yogurt with Granola (6 oz)

190 calories
2 g fat
(1 g saturated)
27 g sugars

Contains less than 1 percent of actual raspberries.

Dannon® la Crème® Peach Yogurt (4 oz)

140 calories
5 g fat
(3 g saturated)
18 g sugars

Stonyfield Farm® Banana Berry Light Smoothie
(1 bottle)

130 calories
0 g fat
20 g sugars

Breakfast Breads

Eat This

Pepperidge Farm® Whole Grain Cinnamon with Raisins Bread
(2 slices)

200 calories
3 g fat (0 g saturated)
280 mg sodium
10 g sugars

Even with butter, two fiber-packed slices are a much healthier option than a frosting-drenched roll.

One English muffin—two halves—has half as many calories as two slices of bread. And whole grain foods keep insulin levels low, so you're less likely to store fat.

Thomas'® 100% Whole Wheat English Muffin

120 calories
1 g fat (0 g saturated)
190 mg sodium

Vitalicious™ AppleBerryBran™ VitaMuffin™ (4 oz)

200 calories
0 g fat
280 mg sodium
20 g sugars

VitaMuffins™ (vitalicious.com) contain 100 percent of your recommended intake of several important nutrients, including vitamins A, B6, B12, C, D, and E.

LUNA® Berry Pomegranate Tea Cake

140 calories
1.5 g fat
(.5 g saturated)
140 mg sodium
12 g sugars

This PopTart replacement gets its sweetness from blueberries and pomegranate puree, and its nutritional punch from green tea extracts and flaxseed.

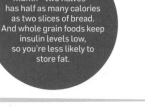
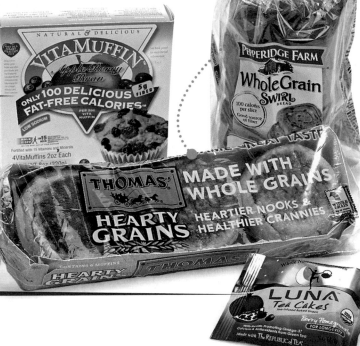

200

Not That!

Thomas' Hearty Grains Oatmeal & Honey Bagel

290 calories
2 g fat (.5 g saturated)
460 mg sodium
58 g carbs

According to the *Journal of the American Medical Association*, when people on low-fat diets replaced just 10 percent of their carbohydrate intake with protein, they decreased their blood pressure, triglycerides, and LDL (bad) cholesterol—reducing heart disease risk by 13 percent. That's the equivalent of trading 60 grams (g) of carbohydrates—about the amount in one bagel—for two servings of lean meat.

Hostess® Blueberry Mini Muffins

(1 pouch)

250 calories
13 g fat
(2.5 saturated)
160 mg sodium
17 g sugars

Kellogg's® Pop Tarts® Frosted Strawberry

(1 pastry)

200 calories
5 g fat
(1 g saturated)
170 mg sodium
19 g sugars

Pillsbury® Cinnamon Rolls

(1 roll)

150 calories
5 g fat
(1.5 g saturated;
2 g trans fat)
350 mg sodium
10 g sugars

This iced roll contains partially hydrogenated oils. Good luck eating just one!

Breakfast Sides

Eat This

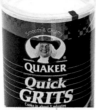

Oscar Mayer® America's Favorite Bacon
(2 slices)

70 calories
6 g fat (2 g saturated)
290 mg sodium

Whole large egg (1)

70 calories
5 g fat (1.5 g saturated)
70 mg sodium

Yolking your diet could rein in your appetite. St. Louis University scientists found that people who eat eggs as part of their breakfast consume fewer calories the rest of the day than those who skip the eggs.

Quaker® Quick Grits
(½ cup uncooked)

260 calories
1 g fat (0 g saturated)
0 g sodium

This creamy Southern staple makes a good stand-in for breakfast potatoes, as long as you take it easy on the butter and cheese.

Al Fresco® Apple Maple Chicken Sausage
(2 links)

140 calories
6 g (2 g saturated)
340 mg sodium

All-natural, low-fat, full-flavor sausage with no nitrates.

Banquet® Brown 'N Serve® Turkey Sausage
(3 links)

110 calories
7 g fat (2 g saturated)
390 mg sodium

Not That!

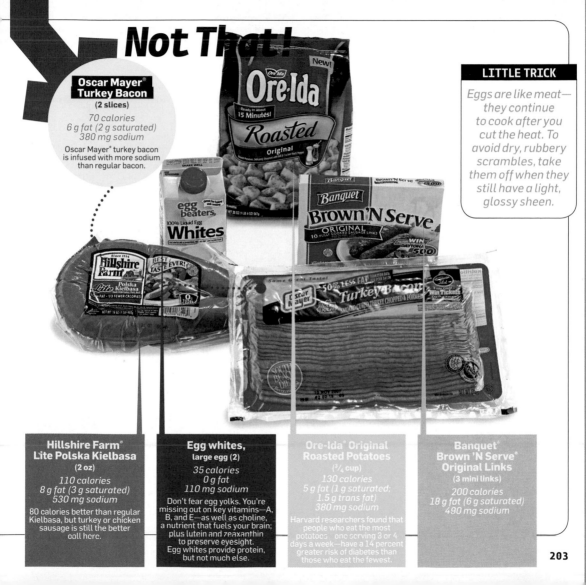

Oscar Mayer® Turkey Bacon
(2 slices)

70 calories
6 g fat (2 g saturated)
380 mg sodium

Oscar Mayer® turkey bacon is infused with more sodium than regular bacon.

LITTLE TRICK

Eggs are like meat— they continue to cook after you cut the heat. To avoid dry, rubbery scrambles, take them off when they still have a light, glossy sheen.

New!

Ore-Ida
Ready In About 15 Minutes!
Roasted
Original

egg beaters
100% Liquid Egg
Whites

Banquet
Brown 'N Serve
ORIGINAL
10 FULLY COOKED SAUSAGE LINKS
WIN DAYTONA 500

Hillshire Farm
Lite
Polska
Kielbasa
FAT • 1/3 FEWER CALORIES

-50% LESS FAT
Turkey Bacon

Hillshire Farm® Lite Polska Kielbasa
(2 oz)

110 calories
8 g fat (3 g saturated)
530 mg sodium

80 calories better than regular Kielbasa, but turkey or chicken sausage is still the better call here.

Egg whites,
large egg (2)

35 calories
0 g fat
110 mg sodium

Don't fear egg yolks. You're missing out on key vitamins—A, B, and E—as well as choline, a nutrient that fuels your brain; plus lutein and zeaxanthin to preserve eyesight. Egg whites provide protein, but not much else.

Ore-Ida® Original Roasted Potatoes
($^3/_4$ cup)

130 calories
5 g fat (1 g saturated; 1.5 g trans fat)
380 mg sodium

Harvard researchers found that people who eat the most potatoes—one serving 3 or 4 days a week—have a 14 percent greater risk of diabetes than those who eat the fewest.

Banquet® Brown 'N Serve® Original Links
(3 mini links)

200 calories
18 g fat (6 g saturated)
490 mg sodium

Breakfast Condiments
Eat This

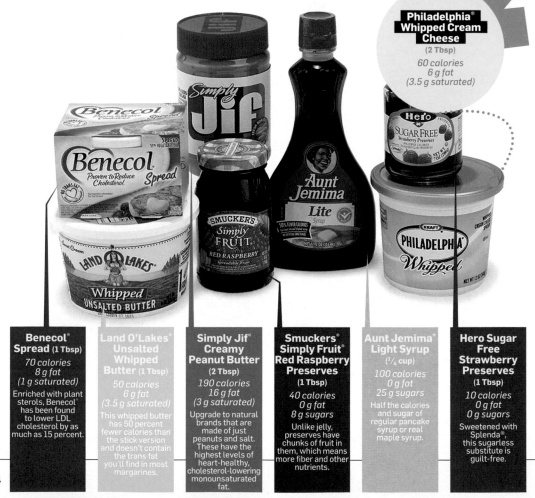

Philadelphia® Whipped Cream Cheese
(2 Tbsp)
60 calories
6 g fat
(3.5 g saturated)

Benecol® Spread (1 Tbsp)
70 calories
8 g fat
(1 g saturated)
Enriched with plant sterols, Benecol® has been found to lower LDL cholesterol by as much as 15 percent.

Land O'Lakes® Unsalted Whipped Butter (1 Tbsp)
50 calories
6 g fat
(3.5 g saturated)
This whipped butter has 50 percent fewer calories than the stick version and doesn't contain the trans fat you'll find in most margarines.

Simply Jif® Creamy Peanut Butter (2 Tbsp)
190 calories
16 g fat
(3 g saturated)
Upgrade to natural brands that are made of just peanuts and salt. These have the highest levels of heart-healthy, cholesterol-lowering monounsaturated fat.

Smuckers® Simply Fruit® Red Raspberry Preserves (1 Tbsp)
40 calories
0 g fat
8 g sugars
Unlike jelly, preserves have chunks of fruit in them, which means more fiber and other nutrients.

Aunt Jemima® Light Syrup (¼ cup)
100 calories
0 g fat
25 g sugars
Half the calories and sugar of regular pancake syrup or real maple syrup.

Hero Sugar Free Strawberry Preserves (1 Tbsp)
10 calories
0 g fat
0 g sugars
Sweetened with Splenda®, this sugarless substitute is guilt-free.

Not That!

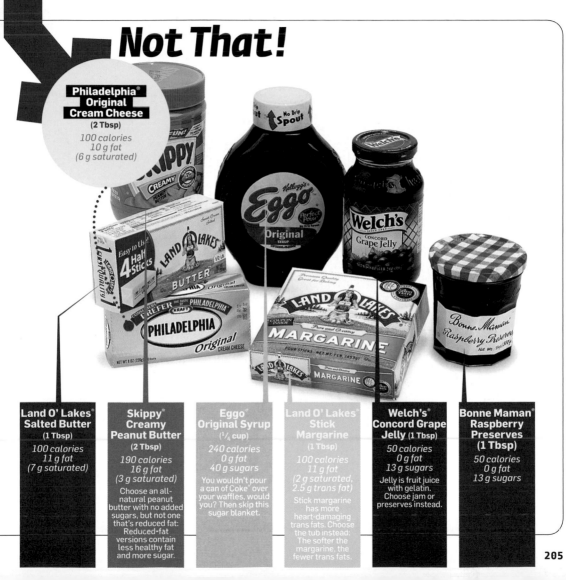

Philadelphia® Original Cream Cheese
(2 Tbsp)
100 calories
10 g fat
(6 g saturated)

Land O' Lakes® Salted Butter
(1 Tbsp)
100 calories
11 g fat
(7 g saturated)

Skippy® Creamy Peanut Butter
(2 Tbsp)
190 calories
16 g fat
(3 g saturated)
Choose an all-natural peanut butter with no added sugars, but not one that's reduced fat: Reduced-fat versions contain less healthy fat and more sugar.

Eggo® Original Syrup
(¹⁄₄ cup)
240 calories
0 g fat
40 g sugars
You wouldn't pour a can of Coke® over your waffles, would you? Then skip this sugar blanket.

Land O' Lakes® Stick Margarine
(1 Tbsp)
100 calories
11 g fat
(2 g saturated, 2.5 g trans fat)
Stick margarine has more heart-damaging trans fats. Choose the tub instead: The softer the margarine, the fewer trans fats.

Welch's® Concord Grape Jelly (1 Tbsp)
50 calories
0 g fat
13 g sugars
Jelly is fruit juice with gelatin. Choose jam or preserves instead.

Bonne Maman® Raspberry Preserves
(1 Tbsp)
50 calories
0 g fat
13 g sugars

205

Snacks

Eat This

Researchers at Penn State found that foods that have been puffed with air are better at satisfying hunger than lower-volume foods that pack the same number of calories.

Glenny's® Organic Sea Salt Soy Crisps
(18 g/$\frac{1}{2}$ bag)
80 calories
1.5 g fat (0 saturated)
125 mg sodium

Tostitos® Natural Organic Yellow Corn Tortilla Chips
(6 chips/1 oz)
140 calories
6 g fat
(.5 g saturated)
100 mg sodium

Newman's Own® Butter Flavor Microwave Popcorn
(3.5 cups/1 oz)
130 calories
5 g fat
(2 g saturated)
200 mg sodium

Doritos® Baked! Nacho Cheese Tortilla Chips
(15 chips/1 oz)
120 calories
3.5 g fat
(.5 g saturated)
220 mg sodium

SunChips® Original Multigrain Snacks
(15 chips/1 oz)
140 calories
6 g fat
(1 g saturated)
120 mg sodium

Lay's® Baked! Original Potato Crisps
(11 crisps/1 oz)
120 calories
2 g fat
(0 g saturated)
180 mg sodium

Rold Gold® Honey Wheat Braided Twists Pretzels
(8 pretzels/1 oz)
110 calories
1 g fat
(.5 g saturated)
230 mg sodium

Not That!

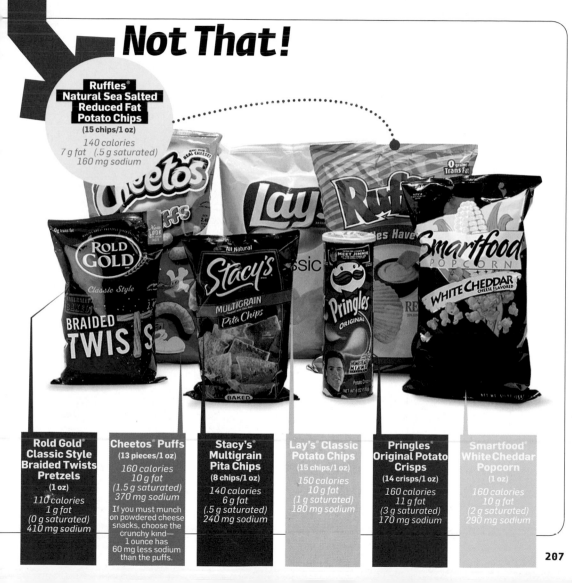

Ruffles® Natural Sea Salted Reduced Fat Potato Chips
(15 chips/1 oz)

140 calories
7 g fat (.5 g saturated)
160 mg sodium

Rold Gold® Classic Style Braided Twists Pretzels
(1 oz)

110 calories
1 g fat
(0 g saturated)
410 mg sodium

Cheetos® Puffs
(13 pieces/1 oz)

160 calories
10 g fat
(1.5 g saturated)
370 mg sodium

If you must munch on powdered cheese snacks, choose the crunchy kind— 1 ounce has 60 mg less sodium than the puffs.

Stacy's® Multigrain Pita Chips
(8 chips/1 oz)

140 calories
6 g fat
(.5 g saturated)
240 mg sodium

Lay's® Classic Potato Chips
(15 chips/1 oz)

150 calories
10 g fat
(1 g saturated)
180 mg sodium

Pringles® Original Potato Crisps
(14 crisps/1 oz)

160 calories
11 g fat
(3 g saturated)
170 mg sodium

Smartfood® White Cheddar Popcorn
(1 oz)

160 calories
10 g fat
(2 g saturated)
290 mg sodium

207

Cookies
Eat This

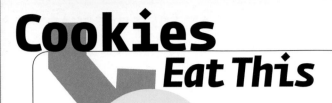

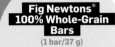

**Fig Newtons®
100% Whole-Grain
Bars**
(1 bar/37 g)
*130 calories
2.5 g fat (0.5 g saturated)
15 g sugars*

**Snackwell's®
Devil's Food Fat Free
Cookie Cakes**
(2 cookies/32 g)
*100 calories
0 g fat
14 g sugars*

**Nilla® Wafers
Reduced Fat**
(8 cookies/30 g)
*110 calories
2 g fat (0 g saturated)
12 g sugars*

Nutter Butters®
(2 cookies/28 g)
*130 calories
6 g fat (1 g saturated)
8 g sugars*

**Snackwell's®
Creme Sandwich
Cookies**
(2 cookies/26 g)
*110 calories
3 g fat (.5 g saturated)
10 g sugars*

**Nabisco®
Ginger Snaps®**
(4 cookies/1 oz)
*120 calories
2.5 g fat (0 g saturated)
11 g sugars*

**Teddy Grahams®
Oatmeal** (24 grahams/30 g)
*130 calories
3.5 g fat (1 g saturated)
8 g sugars*

**Pepperidge Farm®
Chocolate Hazelnut
Pirouettes®**
(2 wafers)
*120 calories
5 g fat (2 g saturated)
13 g sugars*

Not That!

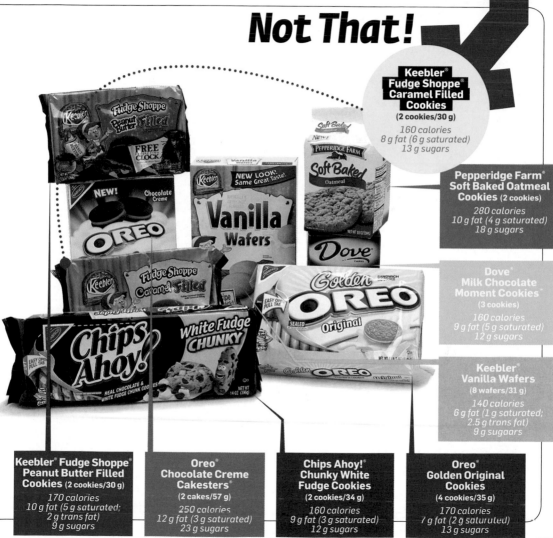

Keebler® Fudge Shoppe® Caramel Filled Cookies
(2 cookies/30 g)

160 calories
8 g fat (6 g saturated)
13 g sugars

Pepperidge Farm® Soft Baked Oatmeal Cookies (2 cookies)

280 calories
10 g fat (4 g saturated)
18 g sugars

Dove® Milk Chocolate Moment Cookies®
(3 cookies)

160 calories
9 g fat (5 g saturated)
12 g sugars

Keebler® Vanilla Wafers
(8 wafers/31 g)

140 calories
6 g fat (1 g saturated;
2.5 g trans fat)
9 g sugaars

Keebler® Fudge Shoppe® Peanut Butter Filled Cookies (2 cookies/30 g)

170 calories
10 g fat (5 g saturated;
2 g trans fat)
9 g sugars

Oreo® Chocolate Creme Cakesters®
(2 cakes/57 g)

250 calories
12 g fat (3 g saturated)
23 g sugars

Chips Ahoy!® Chunky White Fudge Cookies
(2 cookies/34 g)

160 calories
9 g fat (3 g saturated)
12 g sugars

Oreo® Golden Original Cookies
(4 cookies/35 g)

170 calories
7 g fat (2 g saturated)
13 g sugars

Bars

Eat This

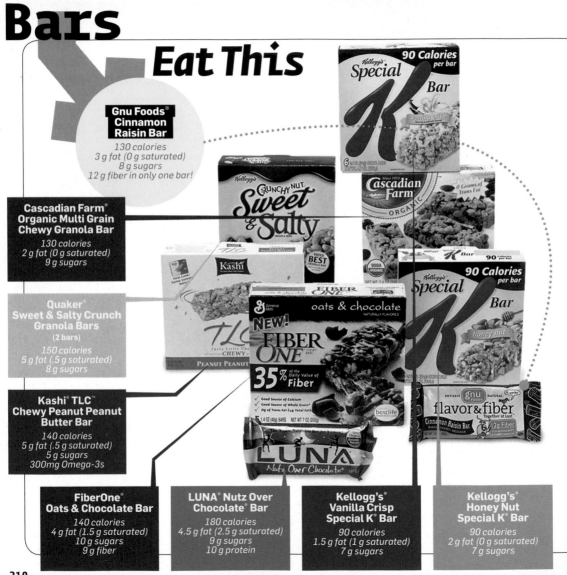

Gnu Foods® Cinnamon Raisin Bar

130 calories
3 g fat (0 g saturated)
8 g sugars
12 g fiber in only one bar!

Cascadian Farm® Organic Multi Grain Chewy Granola Bar

130 calories
2 g fat (0 g saturated)
9 g sugars

Quaker® Sweet & Salty Crunch Granola Bars

(2 bars)

150 calories
5 g fat (.5 g saturated)
8 g sugars

Kashi® TLC™ Chewy Peanut Peanut Butter Bar

140 calories
5 g fat (.5 g saturated)
5 g sugars
300mg Omega-3s

FiberOne® Oats & Chocolate Bar

140 calories
4 g fat (1.5 g saturated)
10 g sugars
9 g fiber

LUNA® Nutz Over Chocolate® Bar

180 calories
4.5 g fat (2.5 g saturated)
9 g sugars
10 g protein

Kellogg's® Vanilla Crisp Special K® Bar

90 calories
1.5 g fat (1 g saturated)
7 g sugars

Kellogg's® Honey Nut Special K® Bar

90 calories
2 g fat (0 g saturated)
7 g sugars

Not That!

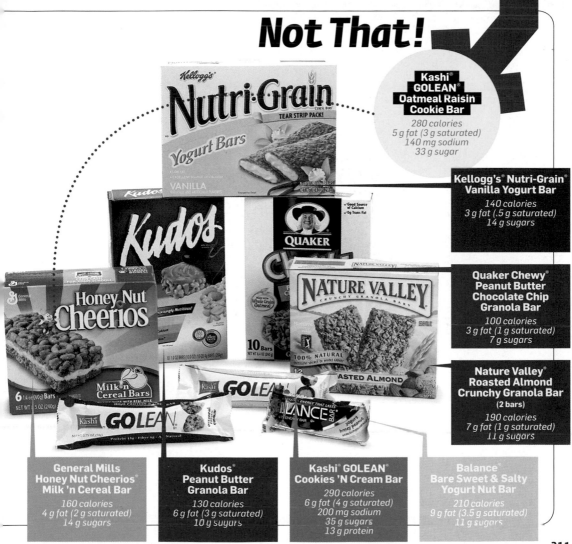

Kashi® GOLEAN® Oatmeal Raisin Cookie Bar

280 calories
5 g fat (3 g saturated)
140 mg sodium
33 g sugar

Kellogg's® Nutri-Grain® Vanilla Yogurt Bar

140 calories
3 g fat (.5 g saturated)
14 g sugars

Quaker Chewy® Peanut Butter Chocolate Chip Granola Bar

100 calories
3 g fat (1 g saturated)
7 g sugars

Nature Valley® Roasted Almond Crunchy Granola Bar (2 bars)

190 calories
7 g fat (1 g saturated)
11 g sugars

General Mills Honey Nut Cheerios® Milk 'n Cereal Bar

160 calories
4 g fat (2 g saturated)
14 g sugars

Kudos® Peanut Butter Granola Bar

130 calories
6 g fat (3 g saturated)
10 g sugars

Kashi® GOLEAN® Cookies 'N Cream Bar

290 calories
6 g fat (4 g saturated)
200 mg sodium
35 g sugars
13 g protein

Balance® Bare Sweet & Salty Yogurt Nut Bar

210 calories
9 g fat (3.5 g saturated)
11 g sugars

211

Dips & Spreads

Eat This

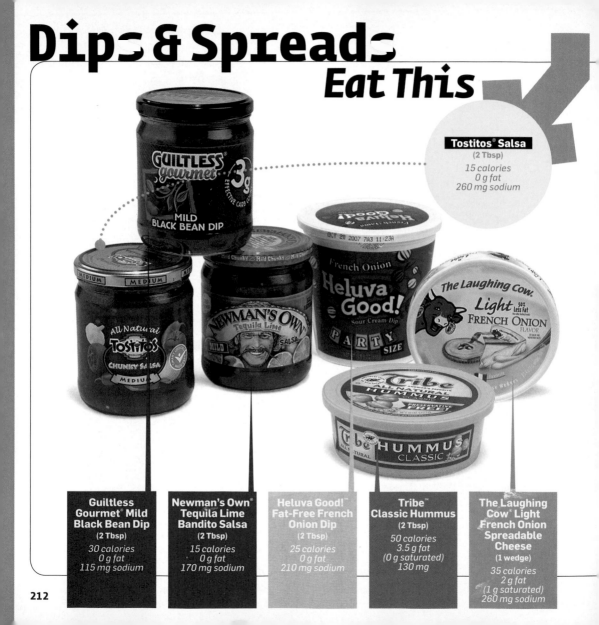

Tostitos® Salsa
(2 Tbsp)
15 calories
0 g fat
260 mg sodium

Guiltless Gourmet® Mild Black Bean Dip
(2 Tbsp)
30 calories
0 g fat
115 mg sodium

Newman's Own® Tequila Lime Bandito Salsa
(2 Tbsp)
15 calories
0 g fat
170 mg sodium

Heluva Good!™ Fat-Free French Onion Dip
(2 Tbsp)
25 calories
0 g fat
210 mg sodium

Tribe™ Classic Hummus
(2 Tbsp)
50 calories
3.5 g fat
(0 g saturated)
130 mg

The Laughing Cow® Light French Onion Spreadable Cheese
(1 wedge)
35 calories
2 g fat
(1 g saturated)
260 mg sodium

Not That!

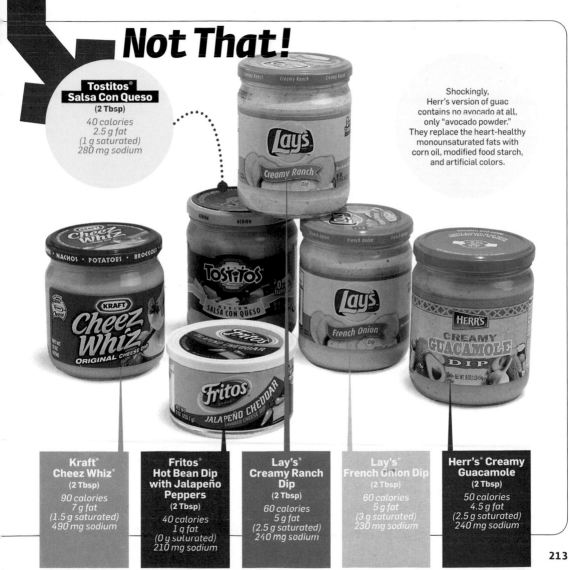

Tostitos® Salsa Con Queso
(2 Tbsp)

40 calories
2.5 g fat
(1 g saturated)
280 mg sodium

Shockingly, Herr's version of guac contains no avocado at all, only "avocado powder." They replace the heart-healthy monounsaturated fats with corn oil, modified food starch, and artificial colors.

Kraft® Cheez Whiz®
(2 Tbsp)

90 calories
7 g fat
(1.5 g saturated)
490 mg sodium

Fritos® Hot Bean Dip with Jalapeño Peppers
(2 Tbsp)

40 calories
1 g fat
(0 g saturated)
210 mg sodium

Lay's® Creamy Ranch Dip
(2 Tbsp)

60 calories
5 g fat
(2.5 g saturated)
240 mg sodium

Lay's® French Onion Dip
(2 Tbsp)

60 calories
5 g fat
(3 g saturated)
230 mg sodium

Herr's® Creamy Guacamole
(2 Tbsp)

50 calories
4.5 g fat
(2.5 g saturated)
240 mg sodium

Salad Dressings
Eat This

South Beach Diet™ Ranch Dressing
(2 Tbsp)

70 calories
7 g fat (1 g saturated)
300 mg sodium

Half the calories and fat of the leading brand.

Newman's Own® Lighten Up!™ Italian Dressing (2 Tbsp)

60 calories
6 g fat (1 g saturated)
260 mg sodium

People whose diets include as much as 2 ounces of olive oil a day have an 82 percent lower risk of having a fatal first heart attack than those who consume little or none.

Wish-Bone® Salad Spritzers™ Caesar Delight™ Vinaigrette (10 sprays)

15 calories
1 g fat (0 g saturated)
85 mg sodium

With less than 2 calories per spray, feel free to indulge. You can afford to have an itchy trigger finger.

Ken's Steak House® Lite Asian Sesame with Ginger & Soy Dressing (2 Tbsp)

70 calories
4 g fat (0 g saturated)
450 mg sodium

Spiked with soy, lime juice, and orange juice, this dressing has almost a third of the fat of Ken's® regular dressing but doesn't sacrifice flavor.

Annie's® Naturals Balsamic Vinaigrette Dressing (2 Tbsp)

100 calories
10 g fat (1 g saturated)
75 mg sodium

No high-fructose corn syrup—just canola oil, balsamic vinegar, honey, organic mustard, and sea salt.

Not That!

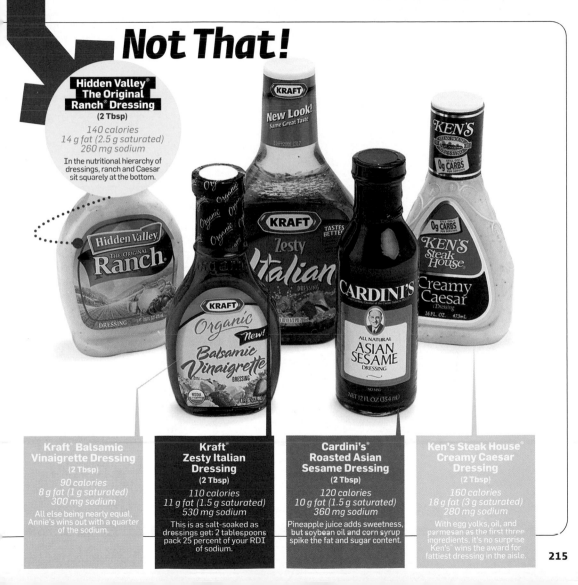

Hidden Valley® The Original Ranch® Dressing
(2 Tbsp)

140 calories
14 g fat (2.5 g saturated)
260 mg sodium

In the nutritional hierarchy of dressings, ranch and Caesar sit squarely at the bottom.

Kraft® Balsamic Vinaigrette Dressing
(2 Tbsp)

90 calories
8 g fat (1 g saturated)
300 mg sodium

All else being nearly equal, Annie's wins out with a quarter of the sodium.

Kraft® Zesty Italian Dressing
(2 Tbsp)

110 calories
11 g fat (1.5 g saturated)
530 mg sodium

This is as salt-soaked as dressings get: 2 tablespoons pack 25 percent of your RDI of sodium.

Cardini's® Roasted Asian Sesame Dressing
(2 Tbsp)

120 calories
10 g fat (1.5 g saturated)
360 mg sodium

Pineapple juice adds sweetness, but soybean oil and corn syrup spike the fat and sugar content.

Ken's Steak House® Creamy Caesar Dressing
(2 Tbsp)

160 calories
18 g fat (3 g saturated)
280 mg sodium

With egg yolks, oil, and parmesan as the first three ingredients, it's no surprise Ken's® wins the award for fattiest dressing in the aisle.

215

Crackers

Eat This

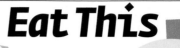

**Keebler®
Cinnamon Crisp®
Low-Fat Grahams**
(8 pieces/28 g)

*110 calories
1.5 g fat
(0 g saturated)
140 mg sodium*

**Carr's®
Table Water® Crackers**
(4 crackers/15 g)

*60 calories
.5 g fat (.5 g saturated)
40 mg sodium*

**Premium™
Low Sodium Saltines**
(10 crackers)

*120 calories
3 g fat (0 g saturated)
50 mg sodium*

**Triscuit®
Reduced Fat**
(7 crackers/29 g)

*120 calories
3 g fat (0 g saturated)
160 mg sodium*

**Pepperidge Farm®
Goldfish® Cheddar
Crackers**
(55 pieces)

*140 calories
5 g fat (1 g saturated)
250 mg sodium*

Not That!

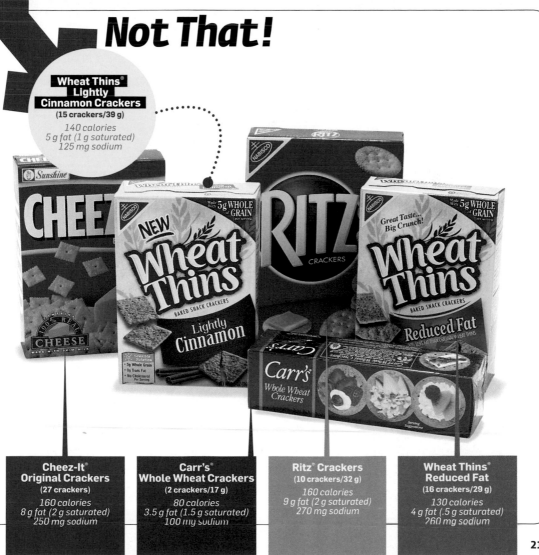

Wheat Thins® Lightly Cinnamon Crackers
(15 crackers/39 g)

140 calories
5 g fat (1 g saturated)
125 mg sodium

Cheez-It® Original Crackers
(27 crackers)

160 calories
8 g fat (2 g saturated)
250 mg sodium

Carr's® Whole Wheat Crackers
(2 crackers/17 g)

80 calories
3.5 g fat (1.5 g saturated)
100 mg sodium

Ritz® Crackers
(10 crackers/32 g)

160 calories
9 g fat (2 g saturated)
270 mg sodium

Wheat Thins® Reduced Fat
(16 crackers/29 g)

130 calories
4 g fat (.5 g saturated)
260 mg sodium

Trail Mix, Dried Fruit,
Eat This

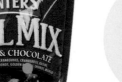

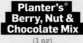

Planter's® Berry, Nut & Chocolate Mix

(1 oz)

120 calories
5 g fat (1 g saturated)
16 g sugars

A Purdue University study found that those who munched on nuts high in monounsaturated fat felt full 90 minutes longer than those who snacked on low-fat foods like rice cakes (or 100 calorie packs)

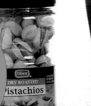

Sun-Maid® Dried Apricots (¼ cup)

100 calories
0 g fat
21 g sugars

Half a cup of dried apricots offers beta carotene, calcium, potassium, and vitamin E, with 3 grams of fiber.

Pistachios, raw (1 oz)

160 calories
13 g fat (1.5 g saturated)
2 g sugars

Phytosterols in pistachios can provide a 10-point drop in triglycerides and a 16-point decline in LDL (bad) cholesterol.

Woodstock Farms Natural Goji Berries (¼ cup)

112 calories
1.4 g fat (0 g saturated)
4 g sugars

Goji berries have one of the highest antioxidant levels of any fruit, according to Tufts University researchers.

Fisher® Nature's™ Nut Mix (1 oz)

150 calories
12 g fat (1 g saturated)
5 g sugars

No sugary or salty dusting. Just a blend of walnuts, almonds, pecans, hazelnuts, raisins, and dried cranberries.

Blue Diamond® Whole Natural Almonds (1 oz)

170 calories
14 g fat (1 g saturated)
0 g sugars

An ounce of almonds provides half the vitamin E you need in a day.

and Mixed Nuts
Not That!

AT THE SUPERMARKET

● Harvard researchers found that men who replaced 127 calories of carbohydrates— that's about 14 Baked Lay's® potato chips— with 1 ounce of nuts decreased their risk of heart disease by 30 percent.

Planter's® Nut & Chocolate Trail Mix
(1 oz)

160 calories
10 g fat (2.5 g saturated)
13 g sugars

Sun-Maid® Vanilla Yogurt Raisins
(¼ cup/30 g)

130 calories
5 g fat
(4 g saturated)
19 g sugars

The "yogurt" makes these closer to candy than a healthy snack.

Planter's® Dry Roasted Peanuts (1 oz)

170 calories
14 g fat
(2 g saturated)
2 g sugars

Peanuts are the low nut on the nutritional totem pole, with a fraction of the antioxidants found in pistachios and walnuts.

Stoneridge Orchards Whole Dried Strawberries

140 calories
0 g fat
32 g sugars

These strawberries are mixed with high-fructose corn syrup. Go fresh instead.

Craisins® Original Sweetened Dried Cranberries
(⅓ cup/42 g)

138 calories
0.5 g fat
30 g sugars

Just as they do with their juice, Ocean Spray® counteracts the cranberry tartness with loads of sugar.

219

Soups

Eat This

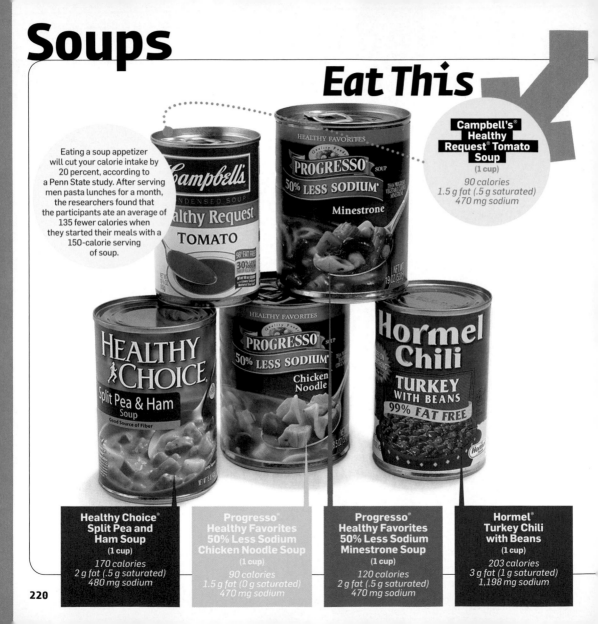

Eating a soup appetizer will cut your calorie intake by 20 percent, according to a Penn State study. After serving men pasta lunches for a month, the researchers found that the participants ate an average of 135 fewer calories when they started their meals with a 150-calorie serving of soup.

Campbell's® Healthy Request® Tomato Soup
(1 cup)
90 calories
1.5 g fat (.5 g saturated)
470 mg sodium

Healthy Choice® Split Pea and Ham Soup
(1 cup)
170 calories
2 g fat (.5 g saturated)
480 mg sodium

Progresso® Healthy Favorites 50% Less Sodium Chicken Noodle Soup
(1 cup)
90 calories
1.5 g fat (0 g saturated)
470 mg sodium

Progresso® Healthy Favorites 50% Less Sodium Minestrone Soup
(1 cup)
120 calories
2 g fat (.5 g saturated)
470 mg sodium

Hormel® Turkey Chili with Beans
(1 cup)
203 calories
3 g fat (1 g saturated)
1,198 mg sodium

Not That!

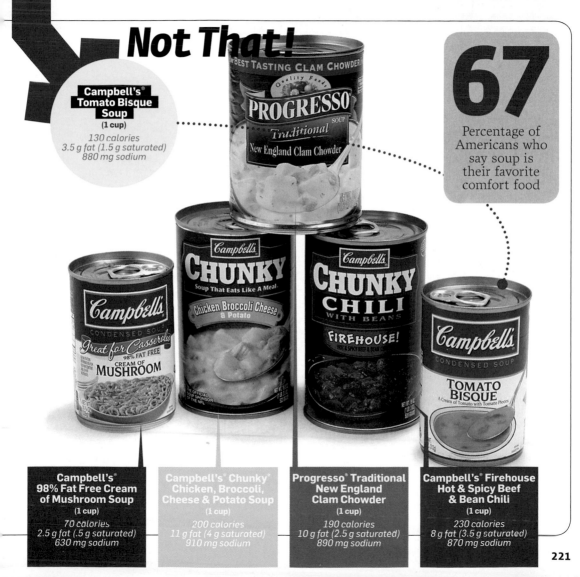

**Campbell's®
Tomato Bisque
Soup**
(1 cup)

*130 calories
3.5 g fat (1.5 g saturated)
880 mg sodium*

67

Percentage of
Americans who
say soup is
their favorite
comfort food

**Campbell's®
98% Fat Free Cream
of Mushroom Soup**
(1 cup)

*70 calories
2.5 g fat (.5 g saturated)
630 mg sodium*

**Campbell's® Chunky®
Chicken, Broccoli,
Cheese & Potato Soup**
(1 cup)

*200 calories
11 g fat (4 g saturated)
910 mg sodium*

**Progresso® Traditional
New England
Clam Chowder**
(1 cup)

*190 calories
10 g fat (2.5 g saturated)
890 mg sodium*

**Campbell's® Firehouse
Hot & Spicy Beef
& Bean Chili**
(1 cup)

*230 calories
8 g fat (3.5 g saturated)
870 mg sodium*

221

Ice Cream

Eat This

**Breyers®
Creamery Style
Cookies & Cream**
(1/2 cup)
140 calories
5 g fat
(3 g saturated)
16 g sugars

Half the saturated fat of Dreyer's®/Edy's® Mint Chocolate Chip, and at least three fewer grams of fat than their Cookies & Cream and Chocolate Chip flavors.

Häagen-Dazs® Low Fat Chocolate Sorbet (1/2 cup)

130 calories
.5 g fat (0 g saturated)
20 g sugar

More sugar and 40 more calories than Turkey Hill® No Sugar Added variety, but when it comes to ice cream, we're willing to sacrifice a few calories for the sake of purity.

Edy's®/Dreyer's® Slow Churned® Rich & Creamy™ Black Cherry Vanilla Swirl Yogurt (1/2 cup)

100 calories
3 g fat (1.5 g saturated)
13 g sugars

Cherry vanilla yogurt with a fraction of the sugar of Ben & Jerry's® Grateful Dead tribute.

Breyers® All Natural Vanilla Fudge Twirl (1/2 cup)

130 calories
6 g fat (4 g saturated)
15 g sugars

A flavor made with refreshingly natural ingredients, composed mostly of milk, cream, sugar, vanilla, and cocoa.

Ben & Jerry's® Berried Treasure Sorbet (1/2 cup)

110 calories
0 g fat 24 g sugars

Premium ice creams and sorbets like Ben & Jerry's® and Häagen-Dazs® often contain up to double the sugar content as brands such as Edy's®/ Dreyer's®, Breyers®, or Turkey Hill®. This swirl also includes real blueberries, blackberries, and lemon puree.

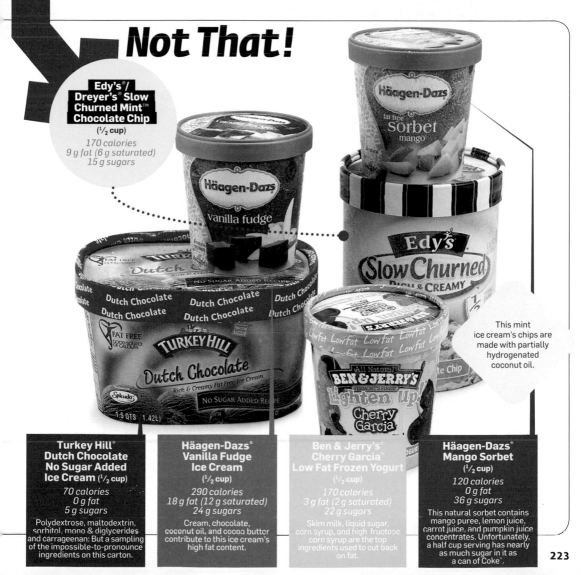

Not That!

Edy's®/ Dreyer's® Slow Churned Mint™ Chocolate Chip
(¹⁄₂ cup)

170 calories
9 g fat (6 g saturated)
15 g sugars

This mint ice cream's chips are made with partially hydrogenated coconut oil.

Turkey Hill® Dutch Chocolate No Sugar Added Ice Cream (¹⁄₂ cup)

70 calories
0 g fat
5 g sugars

Polydextrose, maltodextrin, sorbitol, mono & diglycerides and carrageenan: But a sampling of the impossible-to-pronounce ingredients on this carton.

Häagen-Dazs® Vanilla Fudge Ice Cream (¹⁄₂ cup)

290 calories
18 g fat (12 g saturated)
24 g sugars

Cream, chocolate, coconut oil, and cocoa butter contribute to this ice cream's high fat content.

Ben & Jerry's® Cherry Garcia™ Low Fat Frozen Yogurt (¹⁄₂ cup)

170 calories
3 g fat (2 g saturated)
22 g sugars

Skim milk, liquid sugar, corn syrup, and high fructose corn syrup are the top ingredients used to cut back on fat.

Häagen-Dazs® Mango Sorbet (¹⁄₂ cup)

120 calories
0 g fat
36 g sugars

This natural sorbet contains mango puree, lemon juice, carrot juice, and pumpkin juice concentrates. Unfortunately, a half cup serving has nearly as much sugar in it as a can of Coke®.

223

Frozen Treats

Eat This

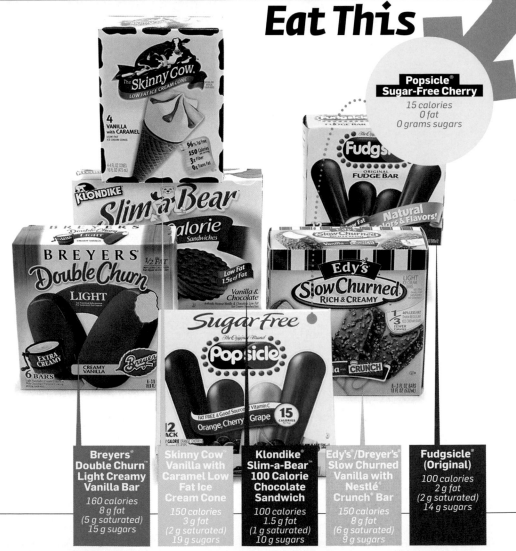

Popsicle® Sugar-Free Cherry
15 calories
0 fat
0 grams sugars

Breyers® Double Churn™ Light Creamy Vanilla Bar
160 calories
8 g fat
(5 g saturated)
15 g sugars

Skinny Cow® Vanilla with Caramel Low Fat Ice Cream Cone
150 calories
3 g fat
(2 g saturated)
19 g sugars

Klondike® Slim-a-Bear™ 100 Calorie Chocolate Sandwich
100 calories
1.5 g fat
(1 g saturated)
10 g sugars

Edy's®/Dreyer's® Slow Churned Vanilla with Nestlé® Crunch® Bar
150 calories
8 g fat
(6 g saturated)
9 g sugars

Fudgsicle® (Original)
100 calories
2 g fat
(2 g saturated)
14 g sugars

Not That!

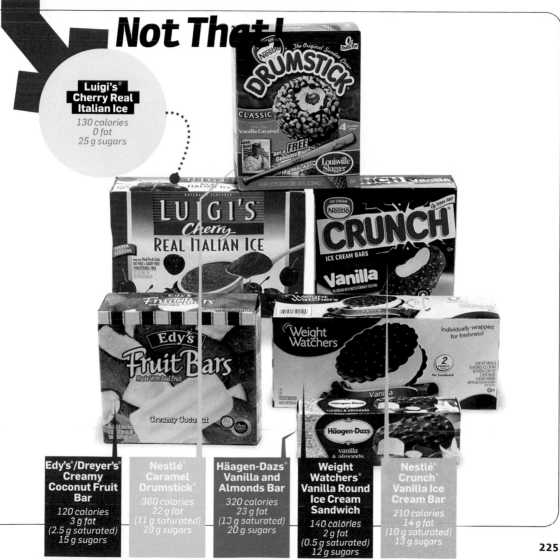

Luigi's® Cherry Real Italian Ice

130 calories
0 fat
25 g sugars

Edy's®/Dreyer's® Creamy Coconut Fruit Bar

120 calories
3 g fat
(2.5 g saturated)
15 g sugars

Nestlé® Caramel Drumstick®

360 calories
22 g fat
(11 g saturated)
29 g sugars

Häagen-Dazs® Vanilla and Almonds Bar

320 calories
23 g fat
(13 g saturated)
20 g sugars

Weight Watchers® Vanilla Round Ice Cream Sandwich

140 calories
2 g fat
(0.5 g saturated)
12 g sugars

Nestlé® Crunch® Vanilla Ice Cream Bar

210 calories
14 g fat
(10 g saturated)
13 g sugars

Indulgences

Live a Little!

What good is losing weight if you're not living well? The fact is, you CAN indulge in ice cream and other frozen desserts, if you do it wisely. Too many of the empty calories we eat come from mindless munching and poor food choices. If, instead, you can nip and tuck calories from your diet by following the guidelines in *Eat This, Not That!*, you'll make room for something that's REALLY a treat. Each of the following tops out at a mere 300 calories.

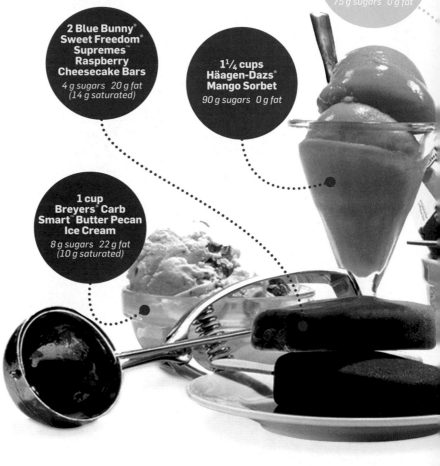

3³⁄₄ Edy's/ Dreyer's Strawberry Fruit Bars
75 g sugars   0 g fat

2 Blue Bunny Sweet Freedom Supremes Raspberry Cheesecake Bars
4 g sugars   20 g fat (14 g saturated)

1¹⁄₄ cups Häagen-Dazs Mango Sorbet
90 g sugars   0 g fat

1 cup Breyers Carb Smart Butter Pecan Ice Cream
8 g sugars   22 g fat (10 g saturated)

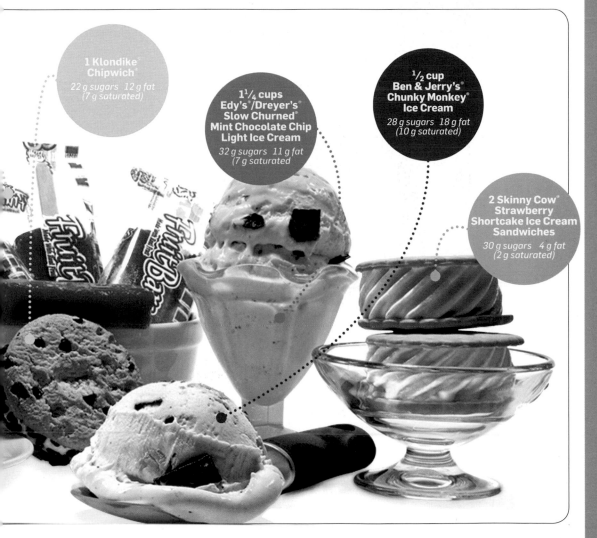

1 Klondike® Chipwich®
22 g sugars 12 g fat
(7 g saturated)

1¼ cups Edy's®/Dreyer's® Slow Churned® Mint Chocolate Chip Light Ice Cream
32 g sugars 11 g fat
(7 g saturated)

½ cup Ben & Jerry's® Chunky Monkey® Ice Cream
28 g sugars 18 g fat
(10 g saturated)

2 Skinny Cow® Strawberry Shortcake Ice Cream Sandwiches
30 g sugars 4 g fat
(2 g saturated)

Frozen Pizza
Eat This

Impressive numbers across the board, including the meager 24 grams of carbs, a result of the ultra thin, crispy crust.

Palermo's® Primo Thin Grilled Chicken Caesar Pizza
(⅓ pizza)
290 calories
12 g fat (6 g saturated)

Lean Pockets® Deli Style Pepperoni Pizza
(1 pocket)
270 calories
7 g fat (2.5 g saturated)
900 mg sodium
In the battle of the unconventional pizza shapes, the nimble pocket trumps the French bread boat every time.

Healthy Choice® Gourmet Supreme Pizza
(1 pizza)
360 calories
4 g fat (1.5 g saturated)
460 mg sodium
The best of the pies from the "healthy" brands.

Not That!

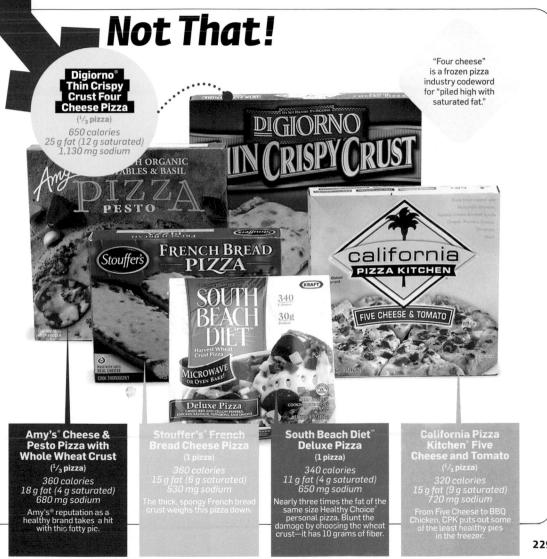

"Four cheese" is a frozen pizza industry codeword for "piled high with saturated fat."

Digiorno® Thin Crispy Crust Four Cheese Pizza
(⅓ pizza)
650 calories
25 g fat (12 g saturated)
1,130 mg sodium

Amy's® Cheese & Pesto Pizza with Whole Wheat Crust
(⅓ pizza)
360 calories
18 g fat (4 g saturated)
680 mg sodium
Amy's® reputation as a healthy brand takes a hit with this fatty pie.

Stouffer's® French Bread Cheese Pizza
(1 pizza)
360 calories
15 g fat (6 g saturated)
530 mg sodium
The thick, spongy French bread crust weighs this pizza down.

South Beach Diet™ Deluxe Pizza
(1 pizza)
340 calories
11 g fat (4 g saturated)
650 mg sodium
Nearly three times the fat of the same size Healthy Choice® personal pizza. Blunt the damage by choosing the wheat crust—it has 10 grams of fiber.

California Pizza Kitchen® Five Cheese and Tomato
(⅓ pizza)
320 calories
15 g fat (9 g saturated)
720 mg sodium
From Five Cheese to BBQ Chicken, CPK puts out some of the least healthy pies in the freezer.

229

Frozen Pasta Entrées

Eat This

**Healthy Choice®
Chicken Broccoli
Alfredo**

*300 calories
5 g fat (2 g saturated)
430 mg sodium*

**Birds Eye® Voila!™ Pesto
Chicken Primavera**

*210 calories
7 g fat (2 g saturated)
590 mg sodium*

Ounce for ounce, Voila!™
makes the healthiest "non-diet"
pastas out there.

**Stouffer's® Lasagna
with Meat & Sauce**

*350 calories
11 g fat (6 g saturated)
930 mg sodium*

They make their pasta from
scratch and form each tray of
lasagna by hand. And it has only
38 grams of carbohydrates.

**Kashi®
Chicken Pasta
Pomodoro**

*280 calories
6 g fat (1.5 g saturated)
470 mg sodium*

Packs an impressive
6 grams of fiber.

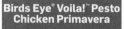

230

Not That!

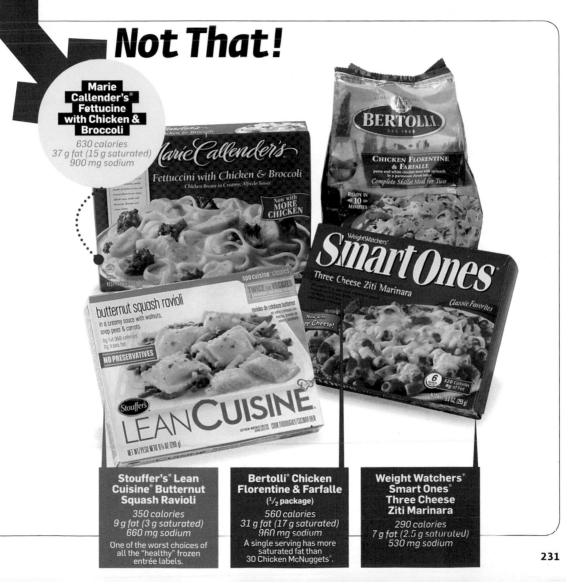

Marie Callender's® Fettucine with Chicken & Broccoli

630 calories
37 g fat (15 g saturated)
900 mg sodium

Stouffer's® Lean Cuisine® Butternut Squash Ravioli

350 calories
9 g fat (3 g saturated)
660 mg sodium

One of the worst choices of all the "healthy" frozen entrée labels.

Bertolli® Chicken Florentine & Farfalle
(¹/₂ **package**)

560 calories
31 g fat (17 g saturated)
960 mg sodium

A single serving has more saturated fat than 30 Chicken McNuggets®.

Weight Watchers® Smart Ones® Three Cheese Ziti Marinara

290 calories
7 g fat (2.5 g saturated)
530 mg sodium

Fish Entrées
Eat This

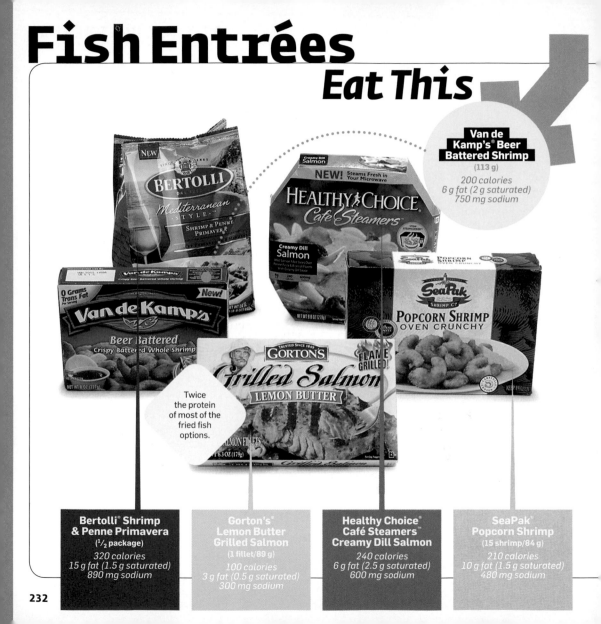

Van de Kamp's® Beer Battered Shrimp
(113 g)
*200 calories
6 g fat (2 g saturated)
750 mg sodium*

Twice the protein of most of the fried fish options.

Bertolli® Shrimp & Penne Primavera
(1/2 package)
*320 calories
15 g fat (1.5 g saturated)
890 mg sodium*

Gorton's® Lemon Butter Grilled Salmon
(1 fillet/89 g)
*100 calories
3 g fat (0.5 g saturated)
300 mg sodium*

Healthy Choice® Café Steamers™ Creamy Dill Salmon
*240 calories
6 g fat (2.5 g saturated)
600 mg sodium*

SeaPak® Popcorn Shrimp
(15 shrimp/84 g)
*210 calories
10 g fat (1.5 g saturated)
480 mg sodium*

Not That!

Gorton's® Beer Batter Shrimp Temptations™
(5 shrimp/99 g)
240 calories
12 g fat (3.5 g saturated)
670 mg sodium

10 CRISPY BATTERED FISH FILLETS

Bertolli® Shrimp Scampi & Linguine
(½ package)
550 calories
23 g fat (10 g saturated)
1,240 mg sodium

Gorton's® Popcorn Shrimp
(20 shrimp/91 g)
240 calories
12 g fat (3.5 g saturated)
830 mg sodium

Gorton's® Crispy Battered Fish Fillets
(2 fillets/104 g)
260 calories
17 g fat (3 g saturated)
770 mg sodium

Stouffer's® Classic Meals Fish Filet
400 calories
16 g fat (4.5 g saturated)
1,050 mg sodium

Chicken Entrées

Eat This

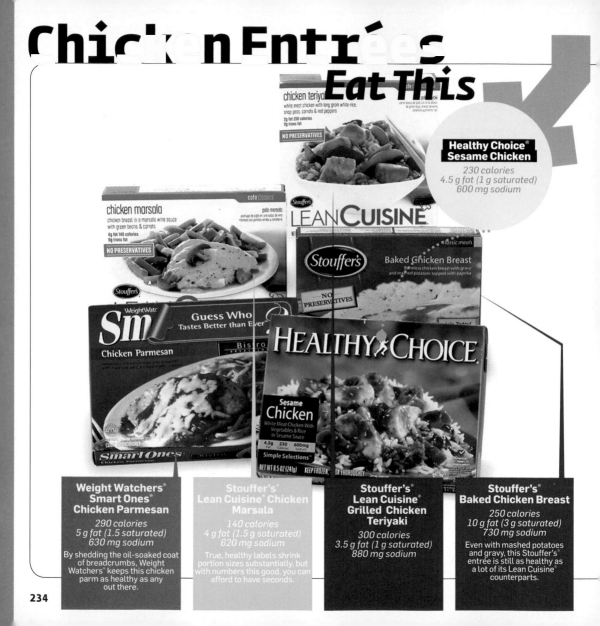

chicken teriyaki
white meat chicken with long grain white rice,
snap peas, carrots & red peppers
2g fat 250 calories
0g trans fat
NO PRESERVATIVES

**Healthy Choice®
Sesame Chicken**

*230 calories
4.5 g fat (1 g saturated)
600 mg sodium*

cafe classics

chicken marsala
chicken breast in a marsala wine sauce
with green beans & carrots
4g fat 140 calories
0g trans fat
NO PRESERVATIVES

pollo marsala

LEAN CUISINE.

Stouffer's

Baked Chicken Breast
Boneless chicken breast with gravy
and mashed potatoes topped with paprika

NO PRESERVATIVES

WeightWatc
Sm
Guess Who
Tastes Better than Ever

Chicken Parmesan

Bisto

Smart Ones
Chicken Parmesan

HEALTHY CHOICE.

Sesame
Chicken
White Meat Chicken With
Vegetables & Rice
In Sesame Sauce

4.5g   230   600mg
Calories   Sodium

Simple Selections™

NET WT 8.5 OZ (241g)   KEEP FROZEN.

**Weight Watchers®
Smart Ones®
Chicken Parmesan**

*290 calories
5 g fat (1.5 saturated)
630 mg sodium*

By shedding the oil-soaked coat
of breadcrumbs, Weight
Watchers™ keeps this chicken
parm as healthy as any
out there.

**Stouffer's®
Lean Cuisine® Chicken
Marsala**

*140 calories
4 g fat (1.5 g saturated)
620 mg sodium*

True, healthy labels shrink
portion sizes substantially, but
with numbers this good, you can
afford to have seconds.

**Stouffer's®
Lean Cuisine®
Grilled Chicken
Teriyaki**

*300 calories
3.5 g fat (1 g saturated)
880 mg sodium*

**Stouffer's®
Baked Chicken Breast**

*250 calories
10 g fat (3 g saturated)
730 mg sodium*

Even with mashed potatoes
and gravy, this Stouffer's®
entrée is still as healthy as
a lot of its Lean Cuisine®
counterparts.

234

Not That!

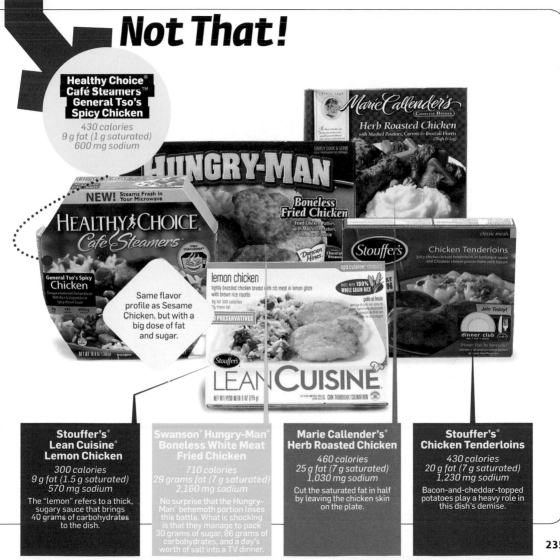

**Healthy Choice®
Café Steamers™
General Tso's
Spicy Chicken**

*430 calories
9 g fat (1 g saturated)
600 mg sodium*

NEW! Steams Fresh in Your Microwave

HEALTHY CHOICE.
Café Steamers™

General Tso's Spicy Chicken

Same flavor profile as Sesame Chicken, but with a big dose of fat and sugar.

HUNGRY-MAN

Boneless Fried Chicken

MarieCallender's
COMPLETE DINNER

Herb Roasted Chicken
with Mashed Potatoes, Carrots & Broccoli Florets
(Thigh & Leg)

SIMPLY COOK & SERVE

Stouffer's
spa cuisine classics

MADE WITH 100% WHOLE GRAIN RICE

lemon chicken
lightly breaded chicken breast with rib meat in lemon glaze with brown rice risotto

NO PRESERVATIVES

Stouffer's
LEANCUISINE

Stouffer's
classic meals

Chicken Tenderloins
Juicy chicken breast tenderloins in barbeque sauce and Cheddar cheese potato bake with bacon

Join Today!
dinner club

**Stouffer's®
Lean Cuisine®
Lemon Chicken**

*300 calories
9 g fat (1.5 g saturated)
570 mg sodium*

The "lemon" refers to a thick, sugary sauce that brings 40 grams of carbohydrates to the dish.

**Swanson® Hungry-Man®
Boneless White Meat
Fried Chicken**

*710 calories
29 grams fat (7 g saturated)
2,160 mg sodium*

No surprise that the Hungry-Man® behemoth portion loses this battle. What is shocking is that they manage to pack 30 grams of sugar, 86 grams of carbohydrates, and a day's worth of salt into a TV dinner.

**Marie Callender's®
Herb Roasted Chicken**

*460 calories
25 g fat (7 g saturated)
1,030 mg sodium*

Cut the saturated fat in half by leaving the chicken skin on the plate.

**Stouffer's®
Chicken Tenderloins**

*430 calories
20 g fat (7 g saturated)
1,230 mg sodium*

Bacon-and-cheddar-topped potatoes play a heavy role in this dish's demise.

Beef Entrées

Eat This

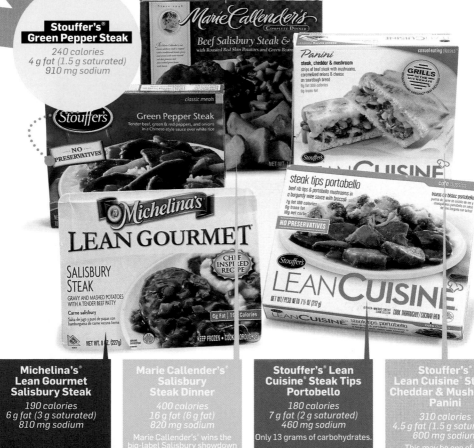

Stouffer's® Green Pepper Steak

240 calories
4 g fat (1.5 g saturated)
910 mg sodium

Marie Callender's
COMPLETE DINNER
Beef Salisbury Steak &
with Roasted Red Skin Potatoes and Green Beans

Stouffer's
Green Pepper Steak
Tender beef, green & red peppers, and onions
in a Chinese-style sauce over white rice
NO PRESERVATIVES

Panini
steak, cheddar & mushroom
strips of beef steak with mushrooms,
caramelized onions & cheese
on sourdough bread

GRILLS
IN THE
MICROWAVE

Michelina's
LEAN GOURMET
SALISBURY STEAK
GRAVY AND MASHED POTATOES
WITH A TENDER BEEF PATTY
Carne salisbury
CHEF INSPIRED RECIPE
NET WT. 8 OZ. (227g)
KEEP FROZEN • COOK THOROUGHLY

steak tips portabello
beef rib tips & portobello mushrooms in
a burgundy wine sauce with broccoli
7g fat 180 calories
6g trans fat
10g net carbs
NO PRESERVATIVES

Stouffer's
LEAN CUISINE
NET WT./PESO NET 10 7½ OZ (212 g)

Michelina's® Lean Gourmet Salisbury Steak

190 calories
6 g fat (3 g saturated)
810 mg sodium

Marie Callender's® Salisbury Steak Dinner

400 calories
16 g fat (6 g fat)
820 mg sodium

Marie Callender's wins the big-label Salisbury showdown in a clean sweep of calories, fat, and sodium.

Stouffer's® Lean Cuisine® Steak Tips Portobello

180 calories
7 g fat (2 g saturated)
460 mg sodium

Only 13 grams of carbohydrates.

Stouffer's® Lean Cuisine® Steak, Cheddar & Mushroom Panini

310 calories
4.5 g fat (1.5 g saturated)
600 mg sodium

This may be one of the healthiest cheesesteaks in America. Pair it with a small salad for a great weekday lunch.

Not That!

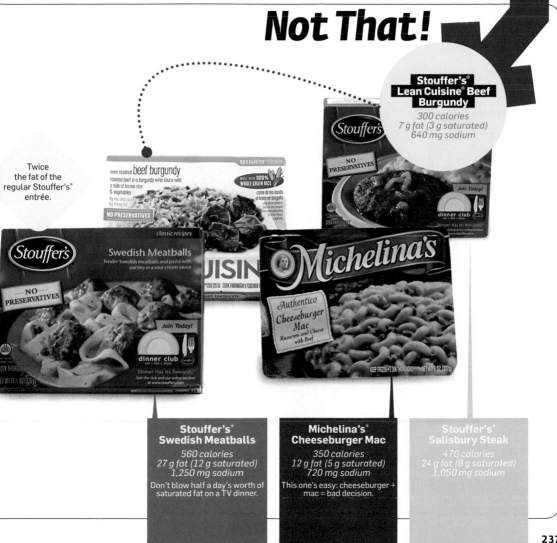

Stouffer's® Lean Cuisine® Beef Burgundy
300 calories
7 g fat (3 g saturated)
640 mg sodium

Twice the fat of the regular Stouffer's® entrée.

Stouffer's® Swedish Meatballs
560 calories
27 g fat (12 g saturated)
1,250 mg sodium
Don't blow half a day's worth of saturated fat on a TV dinner.

Michelina's® Cheeseburger Mac
350 calories
12 g fat (5 g saturated)
720 mg sodium
This one's easy: cheeseburger + mac = bad decision.

Stouffer's® Salisbury Steak
470 calories
24 g fat (8 g saturated)
1,050 mg sodium

Vegetarian Entrées
Eat This

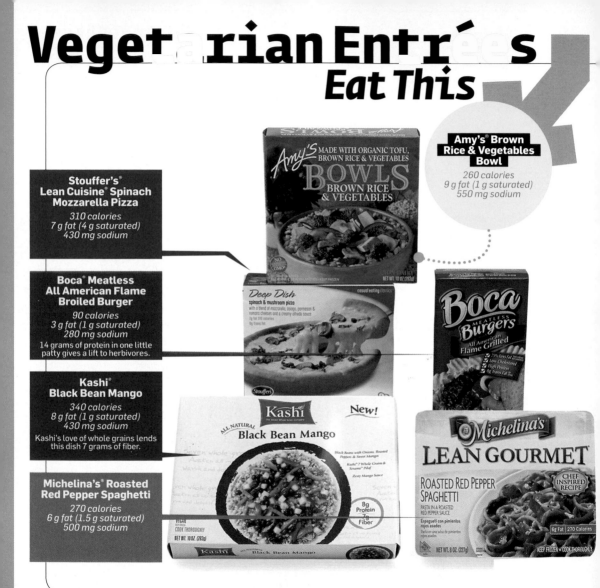

Stouffer's® Lean Cuisine® Spinach Mozzarella Pizza

310 calories
7 g fat (4 g saturated)
430 mg sodium

Amy's® Brown Rice & Vegetables Bowl

260 calories
9 g fat (1 g saturated)
550 mg sodium

Boca® Meatless All American Flame Broiled Burger

90 calories
3 g fat (1 g saturated)
280 mg sodium

14 grams of protein in one little patty gives a lift to herbivores.

Kashi® Black Bean Mango

340 calories
8 g fat (1 g saturated)
430 mg sodium

Kashi's love of whole grains lends this dish 7 grams of fiber.

Michelina's® Roasted Red Pepper Spaghetti

270 calories
6 g fat (1.5 g saturated)
500 mg sodium

238

Not That!

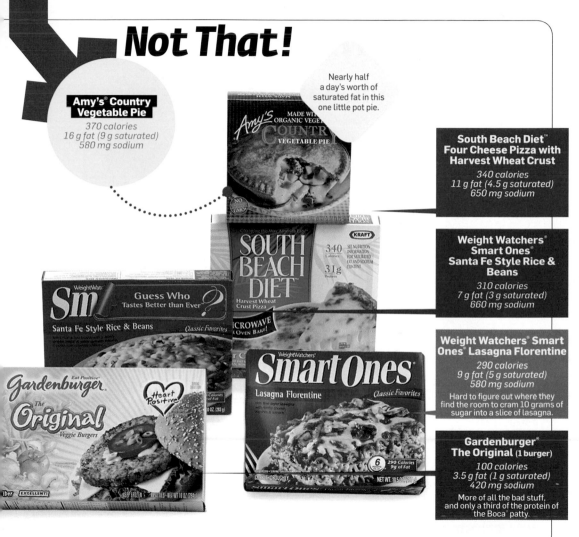

Amy's® Country Vegetable Pie

370 calories
16 g fat (9 g saturated)
580 mg sodium

Nearly half a day's worth of saturated fat in this one little pot pie.

South Beach Diet™ Four Cheese Pizza with Harvest Wheat Crust

340 calories
11 g fat (4.5 g saturated)
650 mg sodium

Weight Watchers® Smart Ones® Santa Fe Style Rice & Beans

310 calories
7 g fat (3 g saturated)
660 mg sodium

Weight Watchers® Smart Ones® Lasagna Florentine

290 calories
9 g fat (5 g saturated)
580 mg sodium

Hard to figure out where they find the room to cram 10 grams of sugar into a slice of lasagna.

Gardenburger® The Original (1 burger)

100 calories
3.5 g fat (1 g saturated)
420 mg sodium

More of all the bad stuff, and only a third of the protein of the Boca® patty.

Breakfast Entrées

Eat This

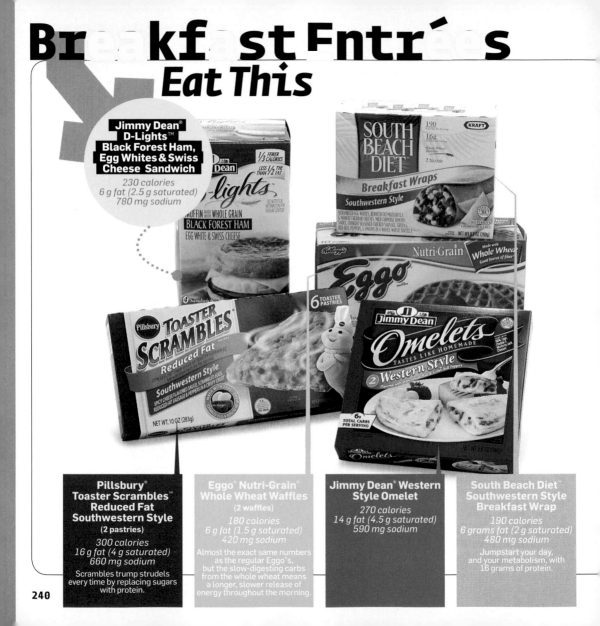

Jimmy Dean® D-Lights™ Black Forest Ham, Egg Whites & Swiss Cheese Sandwich

230 calories
6 g fat (2.5 g saturated)
780 mg sodium

Pillsbury® Toaster Scrambles™ Reduced Fat Southwestern Style
(2 pastries)

300 calories
16 g fat (4 g saturated)
660 mg sodium

Scrambles trump strudels every time by replacing sugars with protein.

Eggo® Nutri-Grain® Whole Wheat Waffles
(2 waffles)

180 calories
6 g fat (1.5 g saturated)
420 mg sodium

Almost the exact same numbers as the regular Eggo's, but the slow-digesting carbs from the whole wheat means a longer, slower release of energy throughout the morning.

Jimmy Dean® Western Style Omelet

270 calories
14 g fat (4.5 g saturated)
590 mg sodium

South Beach Diet™ Southwestern Style Breakfast Wrap

190 calories
6 grams fat (2 g saturated)
480 mg sodium

Jumpstart your day, and your metabolism, with 16 grams of protein.

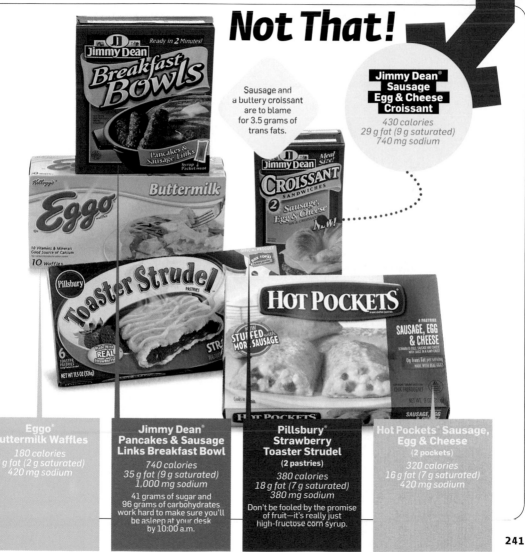

Not That!

Jimmy Dean® Sausage Egg & Cheese Croissant

430 calories
29 g fat (9 g saturated)
740 mg sodium

Sausage and a buttery croissant are to blame for 3.5 grams of trans fats.

Eggo® Buttermilk Waffles

180 calories
6 g fat (2 g saturated)
420 mg sodium

Jimmy Dean® Pancakes & Sausage Links Breakfast Bowl

740 calories
35 g fat (9 g saturated)
1,000 mg sodium

41 grams of sugar and 96 grams of carbohydrates work hard to make sure you'll be asleep at your desk by 10:00 a.m.

Pillsbury® Strawberry Toaster Strudel
(2 pastries)

380 calories
18 g fat (7 g saturated)
380 mg sodium

Don't be fooled by the promise of fruit—it's really just high-fructose corn syrup.

Hot Pockets® Sausage, Egg & Cheese
(2 pockets)

320 calories
16 g fat (7 g saturated)
420 mg sodium

Frozen Snacks
Eat This

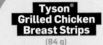

**Tyson®
Grilled Chicken
Breast Strips**
(84 g)

*110 calories
3 g fat (1 g saturated)
480 mg sodium*

Remove the breading and you end up with half the calories and fat, and almost twice the protein in every serving.

**SuperPretzel®
Soft Pretzel
Bites®**
(5 bites/53 g)

*150 calories
0.5 g fat
(0 g saturated)
115 mg sodium*

Nearly a fat-free snack. Pass the spicy mustard, please.

**Amy's®
Spinach Feta
Snacks**
(5 pieces/85 g)

*170 calories
6 g fat
(3 g saturated)
430 mg sodium*

**Tyson®
Buffalo Style
Boneless
Chicken Wyngs**
(3 pieces/85 g)

*142 calories
6.5 g fat
(1 g saturated)
730 mg sodium*

**Ore-Ida®
Steak Fries**
(84 g)

*110 calories
3 g fat
(0.5 g saturated)
330 mg sodium*

**Bagel Bites®
Supreme**
(4 bites/88 g)

*190 calories
5 g fat
(2 g saturated)
560 mg sodium*

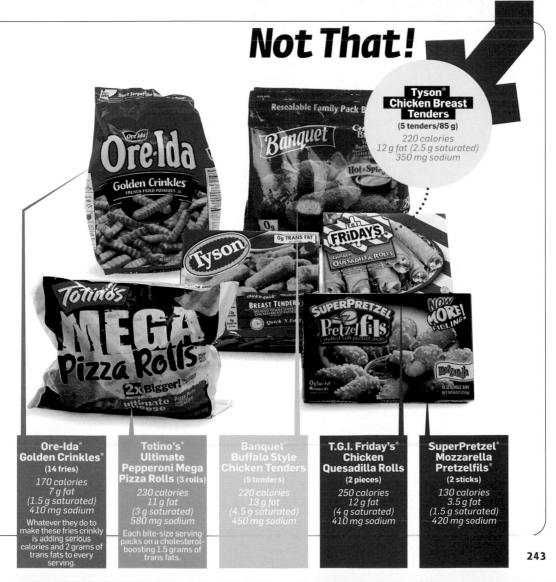

Not That!

Tyson® Chicken Breast Tenders
(5 tenders/85 g)
220 calories
12 g fat (2.5 g saturated)
350 mg sodium

**Ore-Ida®
Golden Crinkles®**
(14 fries)
170 calories
7 g fat
(1.5 g saturated)
410 mg sodium
Whatever they do to make these fries crinkly is adding serious calories and 2 grams of trans fats to every serving.

**Totino's®
Ultimate
Pepperoni Mega
Pizza Rolls (3 rolls)**
230 calories
11 g fat
(3 g saturated)
580 mg sodium
Each bite-size serving packs on a cholesterol-boosting 1.5 grams of trans fats.

**Banquet®
Buffalo Style
Chicken Tenders**
(5 tenders)
220 calories
13 g fat
(4.5 g saturated)
450 mg sodium

**T.G.I. Friday's®
Chicken
Quesadilla Rolls**
(2 pieces)
250 calories
12 g fat
(4 g saturated)
410 mg sodium

**SuperPretzel®
Mozzarella
Pretzelfils®**
(2 sticks)
130 calories
3.5 g fat
(1.5 g saturated)
420 mg sodium

243

Cheeses

Eat This

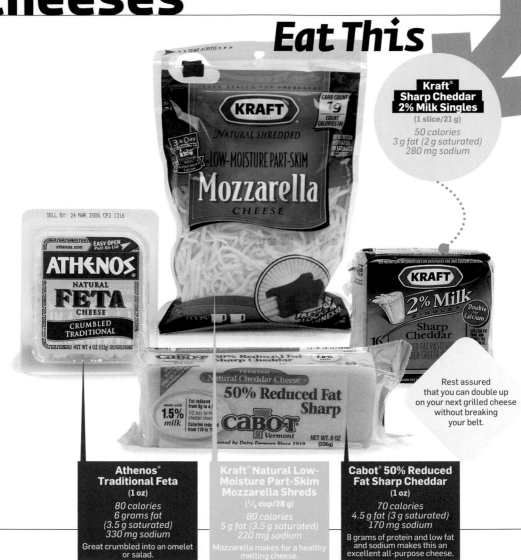

Kraft® Sharp Cheddar 2% Milk Singles
(1 slice/21 g)
50 calories
3 g fat (2 g saturated)
280 mg sodium

KRAFT
NATURAL SHREDDED
LOW-MOISTURE PART-SKIM
Mozzarella
CHEESE

ATHENOS
NATURAL
FETA
CHEESE
CRUMBLED
TRADITIONAL

KRAFT
2% Milk SINGLES
Double the Calcium
Sharp Cheddar

PREMIUM
Natural Cheddar Cheese
50% Reduced Fat Sharp
CaBOT
Vermont
NET WT. 8 OZ (226g)

Rest assured
that you can double up
on your next grilled cheese
without breaking
your belt.

**Athenos®
Traditional Feta**
(1 oz)
80 calories
6 grams fat
(3.5 g saturated)
330 mg sodium
Great crumbled into an omelet
or salad.

**Kraft® Natural Low-
Moisture Part-Skim
Mozzarella Shreds**
(1/4 cup/28 g)
80 calories
5 g fat (3.5 g saturated)
220 mg sodium
Mozzarella makes for a healthy
melting cheese.

**Cabot® 50% Reduced
Fat Sharp Cheddar**
(1 oz)
70 calories
4.5 g fat (3 g saturated)
170 mg sodium
8 grams of protein and low fat
and sodium makes this an
excellent all-purpose cheese.

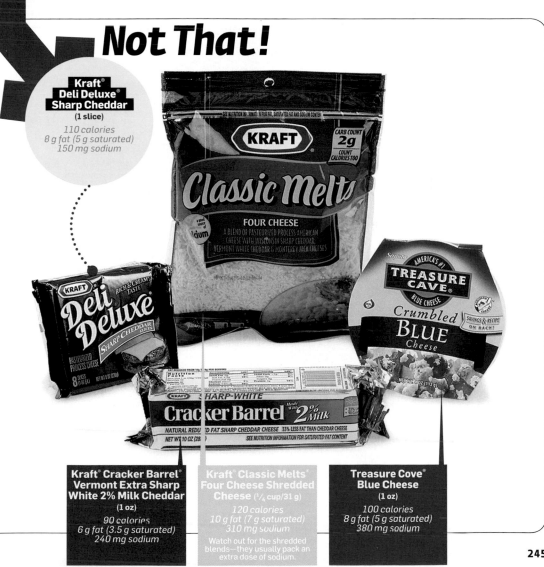

Not That!

Kraft® Deli Deluxe® Sharp Cheddar
(1 slice)

110 calories
8 g fat (5 g saturated)
150 mg sodium

KRAFT

CARB COUNT 2g
COUNT CALORIES TOO

Classic Melts

FOUR CHEESE

A BLEND OF PASTEURIZED PROCESS AMERICAN CHEESE WITH WISCONSIN SHARP CHEDDAR, VERMONT WHITE CHEDDAR & MONTEREY JACK CHEESES

Kraft® Cracker Barrel® Vermont Extra Sharp White 2% Milk Cheddar
(1 oz)

90 calories
6 g fat (3.5 g saturated)
240 mg sodium

Kraft® Classic Melts® Four Cheese Shredded Cheese (¼ cup/31 g)

120 calories
10 g fat (7 g saturated)
310 mg sodium

Watch out for the shredded blends—they usually pack an extra dose of sodium.

Treasure Cove® Blue Cheese
(1 oz)

100 calories
8 g fat (5 g saturated)
380 mg sodium

Deli Meats

Eat This

Unless your supermarket is roasting and slicing meats fresh, this Hormel® line should be your deli meat of choice. It's one of the only products out there produced without nitrates, growth hormones, or other chemicals.

Hormel® Natural Choice® Oven Roasted Deli Turkey
(50 g)

50 calories
1 g fat (0 g saturated)
440 mg sodium

Applegate Farms® Uncured Ham
(2 slices/56 g)

60 calories
1.5 g fat
(0.5 g saturated)
480 mg sodium

No nitrites!

Hillshire Farm® Deli Select® Ultra Thin™ Pastrami
(7 slices)

60 calories
1.5 g fat
(0.5 g saturated)
580 mg sodium

Bumble Bee® Prime Fillet™ Atlantic Salmon
(1/2 can)

80 calories
3.5 g fat
(1 g saturated)
170 mg sodium

1 gram of omega-3 fatty acids in every serving.

Hormel® Natural Choice® Carved Chicken Breast (56 g)

60 calories
1 g fat
(0.5 g saturated)
270 mg sodium

Minimal sodium plus 12 grams of protein. Drop a few chunks onto your next salad.

Hillshire Farm® Deli Select® Ultra Thin™ Roast Beef
(2 oz)

60 calories
2.5 g fat
(1 g saturated)
450 mg sodium

Hormel® Turkey Pepperoni
(17 slices)

70 calories
4 g fat
(1.5 g saturated)
640 mg sodium

Still high in sodium, but a mere 25 percent of the saturated fat of the real stuff.

Not That!

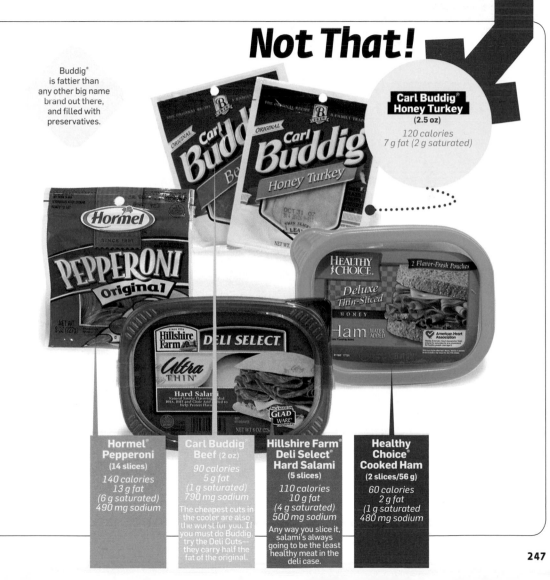

Buddig® is fattier than any other big name brand out there, and filled with preservatives.

Carl Buddig® Honey Turkey
(2.5 oz)

120 calories
7 g fat (2 g saturated)

Hormel® Pepperoni
(14 slices)

140 calories
13 g fat
(6 g saturated)
490 mg sodium

Carl Buddig® Beef (2 oz)

90 calories
5 g fat
(1 g saturated)
790 mg sodium

The cheapest cuts in the cooler are also the worst for you. If you must do Buddig, try the Deli Cuts— they carry half the fat of the original.

Hillshire Farm® Deli Select® Hard Salami
(5 slices)

110 calories
10 g fat
(4 g saturated)
500 mg sodium

Any way you slice it, salami's always going to be the least healthy meat in the deli case.

Healthy Choice® Cooked Ham
(2 slices/56 g)

60 calories
2 g fat
(1 g saturated
480 mg sodium

247

Breads
Eat This

Arnold® Bakery Light 100% Whole Wheat Bread

(2 slices/43 g)

80 calories
0 g fat
5 g fiber

Only 17 grams of carbohydrates and 5 grams of fiber (as much as the Double Fiber). Make this your loaf of choice for sandwiches.

Did You Know?

● White and wheat bread both come from wheat. The only difference is that whole wheat is less refined than white bread. Too bad, since the more man-handled wheat is, the less fibrous—and less filling— it becomes. When choosing a loaf, look for whole wheat bread that con- tains at least 3 grams of fiber per slice.

Pepperidge Farm® Jewish Seeded Rye

(2 slices)

160 calories
2 g fat (0 g saturated)
4 g fiber

Double the fiber by opting for the seeded over the seedless version.

Thomas'® Sahara® Whole Wheat Pita Pocket

130 calories
1 g fat (0 g saturated)
5 g fiber

Pepperidge Farm® Classic 100% Whole Wheat Hamburger Bun

120 calories
2 g fat (0 g saturated)
4 g fiber

More fiber and considerably less sugar than nearly every other roll on the shelves.

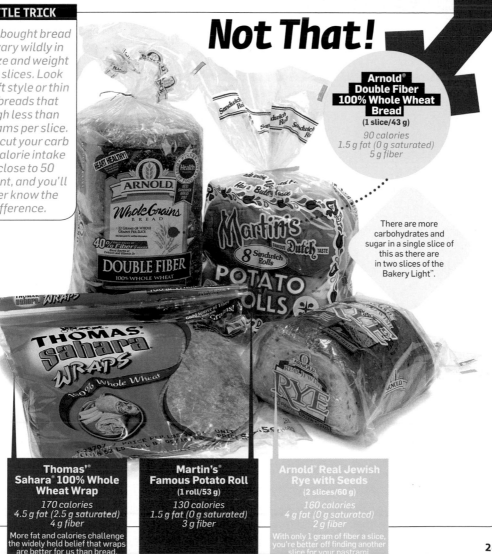

LITTLE TRICK

Store-bought bread can vary wildly in the size and weight of its slices. Look for soft style or thin cut breads that weigh less than 30 grams per slice. You'll cut your carb and calorie intake by close to 50 percent, and you'll never know the difference.

Not That!

**Arnold®
Double Fiber
100% Whole Wheat
Bread**
(1 slice/43 g)

*90 calories
1.5 g fat (0 g saturated)
5 g fiber*

There are more
carbohydrates and
sugar in a single slice of
this as there are
in two slices of the
Bakery Light™.

**Thomas'®
Sahara® 100% Whole
Wheat Wrap**

*170 calories
4.5 g fat (2.5 g saturated)
4 g fiber*

More fat and calories challenge
the widely held belief that wraps
are better for us than bread.

**Martin's®
Famous Potato Roll**
(1 roll/53 g)

*130 calories
1.5 g fat (0 g saturated)
3 g fiber*

**Arnold® Real Jewish
Rye with Seeds**
(2 slices/60 g)

*160 calories
4 g fat (0 g saturated)
2 g fiber*

With only 1 gram of fiber a slice,
you're better off finding another
slice for your pastrami.

249

Condiments

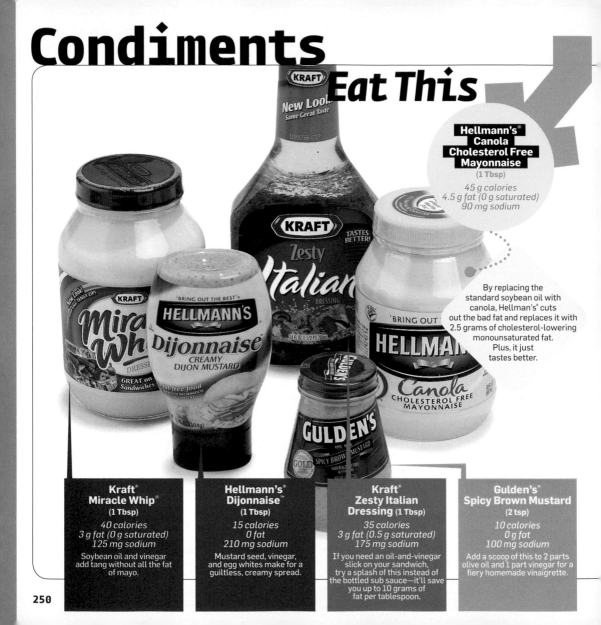

Eat This

**Hellmann's®
Canola
Cholesterol Free
Mayonnaise**
(1 Tbsp)

*45 g calories
4.5 g fat (0 g saturated)
90 mg sodium*

By replacing the standard soybean oil with canola, Hellman's® cuts out the bad fat and replaces it with 2.5 grams of cholesterol-lowering monounsaturated fat. Plus, it just tastes better.

**Kraft®
Miracle Whip®**
(1 Tbsp)

*40 calories
3 g fat (0 g saturated)
125 mg sodium*

Soybean oil and vinegar add tang without all the fat of mayo.

**Hellmann's®
Dijonnaise™**
(1 Tbsp)

*15 calories
0 fat
210 mg sodium*

Mustard seed, vinegar, and egg whites make for a guiltless, creamy spread.

**Kraft®
Zesty Italian
Dressing** (1 Tbsp)

*35 calories
3 g fat (0.5 g saturated)
175 mg sodium*

If you need an oil-and-vinegar slick on your sandwich, try a splash of this instead of the bottled sub sauce—it'll save you up to 10 grams of fat per tablespoon.

**Gulden's®
Spicy Brown Mustard**
(2 tsp)

*10 calories
0 g fat
100 mg sodium*

Add a scoop of this to 2 parts olive oil and 1 part vinegar for a fiery homemade vinaigrette.

Not That!

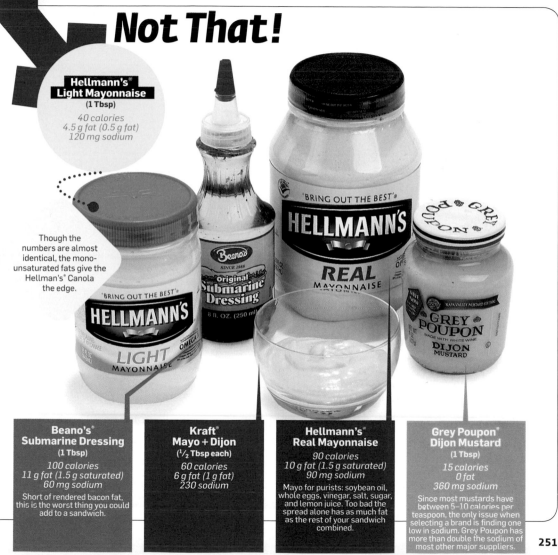

Hellmann's® Light Mayonnaise
(1 Tbsp)

40 calories
4.5 g fat (0.5 g fat)
120 mg sodium

Though the numbers are almost identical, the mono-unsaturated fats give the Hellman's® Canola the edge.

Beano's® Submarine Dressing
(1 Tbsp)

100 calories
11 g fat (1.5 g saturated)
60 mg sodium

Short of rendered bacon fat, this is the worst thing you could add to a sandwich.

Kraft® Mayo + Dijon
(¹/₂ Tbsp each)

60 calories
6 g fat (1 g fat)
230 sodium

Hellmann's® Real Mayonnaise

90 calories
10 g fat (1.5 g saturated)
90 mg sodium

Mayo for purists: soybean oil, whole eggs, vinegar, salt, sugar, and lemon juice. Too bad the spread alone has as much fat as the rest of your sandwich combined.

Grey Poupon® Dijon Mustard
(1 Tbsp)

15 calories
0 fat
360 mg sodium

Since most mustards have between 5–10 calories per teaspoon, the only issue when selecting a brand is finding one low in sodium. Grey Poupon has more than double the sodium of most other major suppliers.

Pasta and Pasta Sauces
Eat This

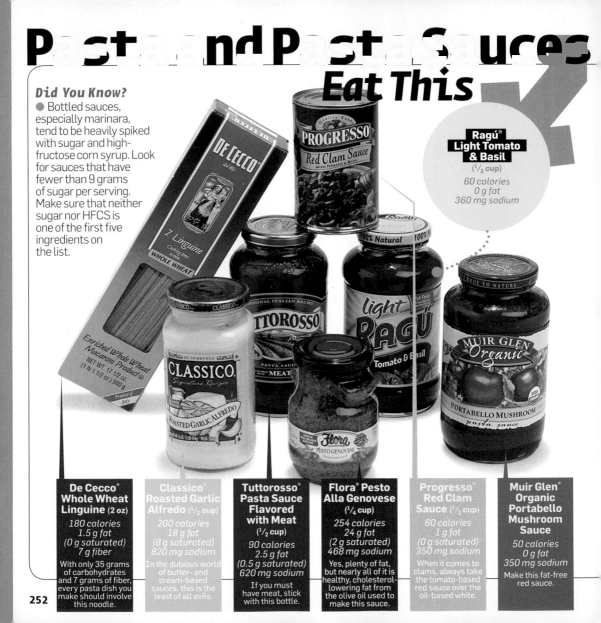

Did You Know?
● Bottled sauces, especially marinara, tend to be heavily spiked with sugar and high-fructose corn syrup. Look for sauces that have fewer than 9 grams of sugar per serving. Make sure that neither sugar nor HFCS is one of the first five ingredients on the list.

**Ragú®
Light Tomato
& Basil**
(½ cup)
*60 calories
0 g fat
360 mg sodium*

**De Cecco®
Whole Wheat
Linguine (2 oz)**
*180 calories
1.5 g fat
(0 g saturated)
7 g fiber*
With only 35 grams of carbohydrates and 7 grams of fiber, every pasta dish you make should involve this noodle.

**Classico®
Roasted Garlic
Alfredo** (½ cup)
*200 calories
18 g fat
(8 g saturated)
820 mg sodium*
In the dubious world of butter- and cream-based sauces, this is the least of all evils.

**Tuttorosso®
Pasta Sauce
Flavored
with Meat**
(½ cup)
*90 calories
2.5 g fat
(0.5 g saturated)
620 mg sodium*
If you must have meat, stick with this bottle.

**Flora® Pesto
Alla Genovese**
(¼ cup)
*254 calories
24 g fat
(2 g saturated)
468 mg sodium*
Yes, plenty of fat, but nearly all of it is healthy, cholesterol-lowering fat from the olive oil used to make this sauce.

**Progresso®
Red Clam
Sauce** (½ cup)
*60 calories
1 g fat
(0 g saturated)
350 mg sodium*
When it comes to clams, always take the tomato-based red sauce over the oil-based white.

**Muir Glen®
Organic
Portabello
Mushroom
Sauce**
*50 calories
0 g fat
350 mg sodium*
Make this fat-free red sauce.

252

Not That!

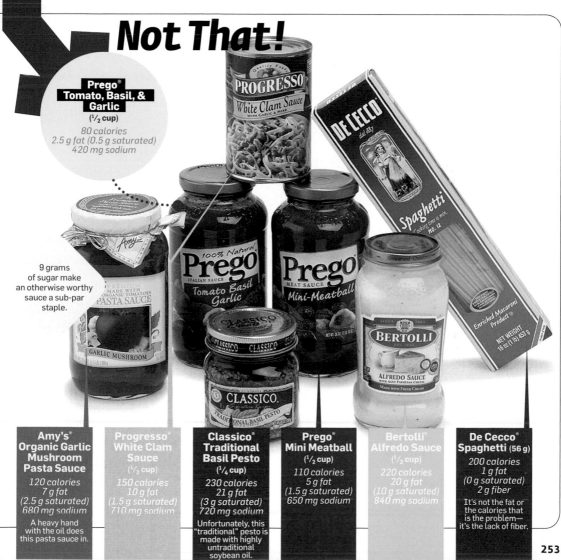

Prego® Tomato, Basil, & Garlic
(½ cup)

80 calories
2.5 g fat (0.5 g saturated)
420 mg sodium

9 grams of sugar make an otherwise worthy sauce a sub-par staple.

Amy's® Organic Garlic Mushroom Pasta Sauce

120 calories
7 g fat
(2.5 g saturated)
680 mg sodium

A heavy hand with the oil does this pasta sauce in.

Progresso® White Clam Sauce
(½ cup)

150 calories
10 g fat
(1.5 g saturated)
710 mg sodium

Classico® Traditional Basil Pesto
(¼ cup)

230 calories
21 g fat
(3 g saturated)
720 mg sodium

Unfortunately, this "traditional" pesto is made with highly untraditional soybean oil.

Prego® Mini Meatball
(½ cup)

110 calories
5 g fat
(1.5 g saturated)
650 mg sodium

Bertolli® Alfredo Sauce
(½ cup)

220 calories
20 g fat
(10 g saturated)
840 mg sodium

De Cecco® Spaghetti (56 g)

200 calories
1 g fat
(0 g saturated)
2 g fiber

It's not the fat or the calories that is the problem—it's the lack of fiber.

253

Chapter 6

EAT
THIS
NOT
THAT!

DRINK THIS, NOT THAT!

Juice

Drink This

*All serving sizes are 8 ounces, unless otherwise noted

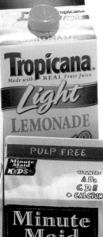

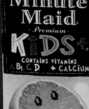

V8® Essential Antioxidants*

50 calories
8 g sugars
470 mg sodium

V8 goes beyond tomatoes, adding spinach, celery, beets, and watercress to the super-charged brew.

Ocean Spray® Light Cranberry Juice Cocktail

40 calories
10 g sugars

Unlike other light juices, they don't stiff you on the fruit here. This has as much cranberry juice (27%) as the original Ocean Spray®, but with a third of the sugar.

Tropicana® Light Lemonade

10 calories
2 g sugars

You lose little actual juice (8% instead of 10% lemon juice), but the high-fructose corn syrup is replaced with Splenda®.

Minute Maid® Kids Multi-Vitamin Orange Juice

120 calories
24 g sugars

OJs are created equal, so look for nutritional bonuses. The juice packs B vitamins essential to energy production.

Tropicana Pure Premium® Orange Juice

110 calories
22 g sugars

You *can* compare apples and oranges, and there's no question which prevails: OJ gets the nod for less sugar and more vitamins, including 250% of your vitamin C.

Ocean Spray® White Grapefruit 100% Juice

90 calories
17 g sugars

As good as juice gets. Make this a familiar face in your fridge.

256

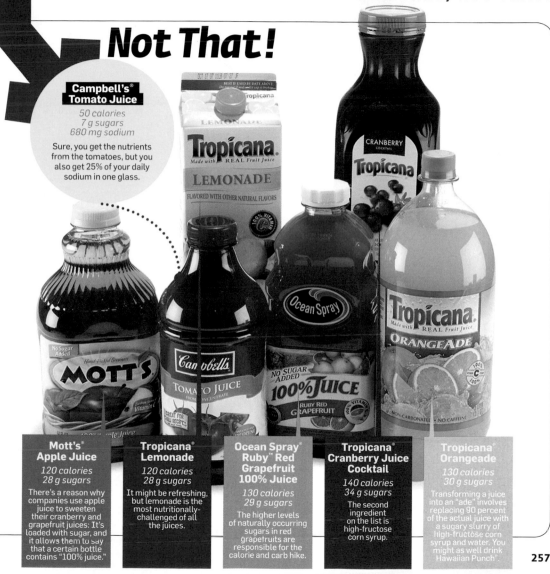

Not That!

Campbell's® Tomato Juice

50 calories
7 g sugars
680 mg sodium

Sure, you get the nutrients from the tomatoes, but you also get 25% of your daily sodium in one glass.

Mott's® Apple Juice

120 calories
28 g sugars

There's a reason why companies use apple juice to sweeten their cranberry and grapefruit juices: It's loaded with sugar, and it allows them to say that a certain bottle contains "100% juice."

Tropicana® Lemonade

120 calories
28 g sugars

It might be refreshing, but lemonade is the most nutritionally-challenged of all the juices.

Ocean Spray® Ruby™ Red Grapefruit 100% Juice

130 calories
29 g sugars

The higher levels of naturally occurring sugars in red grapefruits are responsible for the calorie and carb hike.

Tropicana® Cranberry Juice Cocktail

140 calories
34 g sugars

The second ingredient on the list is high-fructose corn syrup.

Tropicana® Orangeade

130 calories
30 g sugars

Transforming a juice into an "ade" involves replacing 90 percent of the actual juice with a sugary slurry of high-fructose corn syrup and water. You might as well drink Hawaiian Punch®.

Coffee Drinks
Drink This

Dunkin' Donuts®
Vanilla Latte Lite
(10 oz)

80 calories
0 g fat
10 g sugars

Did You Know?

Here's an eye-opener: According to the bean barons at Illy Coffee, a shot of espresso has 35 percent less caffeine than a cup of brewed coffee.

Where does all the sugar come from? Flavor syrups. A single pump adds about 5 grams of sugar to a drink, and with 4–5 pumps in a large latte, the damage multiplies quickly. The simple solution? Ask for sugar-free syrup.

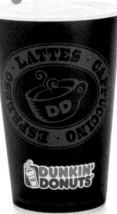

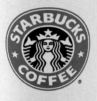

Starbucks®
2% Caffè Mocha
no whip (12 oz)

200 calories
6 g fat
(3.5 g saturated)
24 g sugars

Starbucks®
2% Tazo®
Chai Tea Latte
(12 oz)

180 calories
3 g fat
(2 g saturated)
31 g sugars

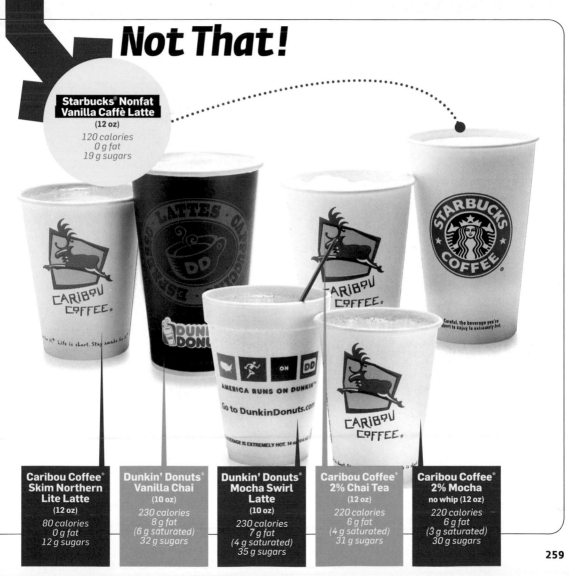

Not That!

Starbucks® Nonfat Vanilla Caffè Latte
(12 oz)
120 calories
0 g fat
19 g sugars

Caribou Coffee® Skim Northern Lite Latte
(12 oz)
80 calories
0 g fat
12 g sugars

Dunkin' Donuts® Vanilla Chai
(10 oz)
230 calories
8 g fat
(6 g saturated)
32 g sugars

Dunkin' Donuts® Mocha Swirl Latte
(10 oz)
230 calories
7 g fat
(4 g saturated)
35 g sugars

Caribou Coffee® 2% Chai Tea
(12 oz)
220 calories
6 g fat
(4 g saturated)
31 g sugars

Caribou Coffee® 2% Mocha
no whip (12 oz)
220 calories
6 g fat
(3 g saturated)
30 g sugars

Iced Coffee Drinks
Drink This

Dunkin' Donuts® Caramel Creme Iced Latte
(16 oz)

260 calories
9 g fat (6 g saturated)
40 g sugars

Ask for half the caramel to cut back on high-fructose corn syrup

AMERICA RUNS ON DUNKIN™

DunkinDonuts.com

Skip the iced coffee before your next public speaking venture: Iced and caffeinated drinks tighten the vocal cords, as do acidic drinks like orange juice. For at least two hours before any nerve-tickling event, stick with liquids at room temperature.

Caribou Coffee® Wild Berry Smoothie
(16 oz)

230 calories
0 g fat
53 g sugars

A lighter hand with the sugar gives Caribou the edge in the blended fruit drinks category.

Not That!

Caribou Coffee® 2% Caramel Cooler
(16 oz)

340 calories
12 g fat (8 g saturated)
50 g sugars

With 50 grams of sugar, this is a caramel milkshake in coffee drag.

Skip the Whip: A scoop of Starbucks' whipped topping adds 70 calories and 7 grams of fat to your drink.

CARIBOU

Starbucks® 2% Iced Dulce de Leche Latte, with whip
(16 oz)

420 calories
16 g fat
(10 g saturated)
52 g sugars

Do you really want to slurp up half a day's worth of saturated fat in a single drink?

Starbucks® Orange Crème Frappuccino®
no whip (16 oz)

320 calories
2 g fat
(0 g saturated)
53 g sugars

Opt for the Orange Mocha Frappuccino® instead and cut more than half the calories and sugar from this Crème.

Dunkin' Donuts® Strawberry Fruit Coolatta®
(16 oz)

290 calories
0 g fat
65 g sugars

Ounce-for-ounce, more sugar than the sweetest soft drinks.

Wake Up and Smell the

From energy drinks to functional waters, the beverage industry is obsessed with bottling America's caffeine addiction. But caffeine content isn't listed on most nutrition labels, so how do you determine how much of a jolt to expect from popular beverages? University of Florida researchers analyzed 36 widely available drinks. We've highlighted the most caffeinated products in five common categories and compared them with our benchmark beverage— a regular black coffee from Dunkin' Donuts®.

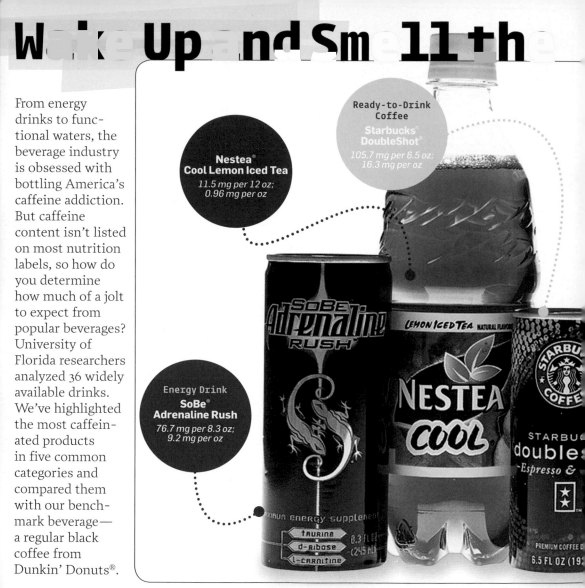

Nestea® Cool Lemon Iced Tea
11.5 mg per 12 oz;
0.96 mg per oz

Ready-to-Drink Coffee
Starbucks® DoubleShot®
105.7 mg per 6.5 oz;
16.3 mg per oz

Energy Drink
SoBe® Adrenaline Rush
76.7 mg per 8.3 oz;
9.2 mg per oz

Caffeine

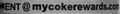
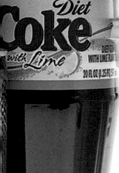

Diet Soda
Diet Coke® with Lime
39.6 mg per 12 oz; 3.3 mg per oz

Black Coffee
Dunkin' Donuts® Regular Coffee
143 mg per 16 oz; 8.9 mg per oz

Regular Soda
Mountain Dew®
45.4 mg per 12 oz; 3.8 mg per oz

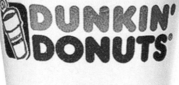

Children's Drinks
Drink This

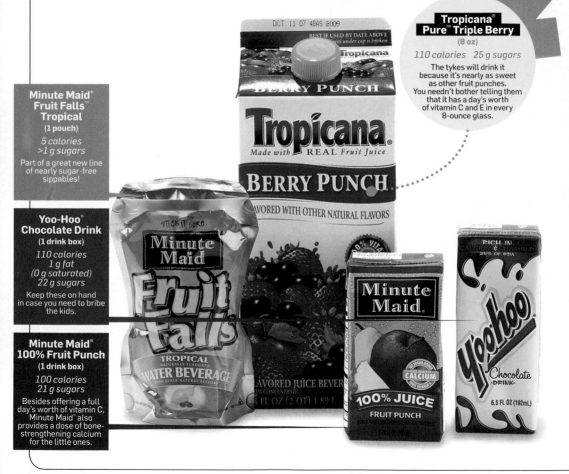

Minute Maid® Fruit Falls™ Tropical
(1 pouch)
5 calories
>1 g sugars
Part of a great new line of nearly sugar-free sippables!

Yoo-Hoo® Chocolate Drink
(1 drink box)
110 calories
1 g fat
(0 g saturated)
22 g sugars
Keep these on hand in case you need to bribe the kids.

Minute Maid® 100% Fruit Punch
(1 drink box)
100 calories
21 g sugars
Besides offering a full day's worth of vitamin C, Minute Maid® also provides a dose of bone-strengthening calcium for the little ones.

Tropicana® Pure™ Triple Berry
(8 oz)
110 calories   25 g sugars
The tykes will drink it because it's nearly as sweet as other fruit punches. You needn't bother telling them that it has a day's worth of vitamin C and E in every 8-ounce glass.

Not That!

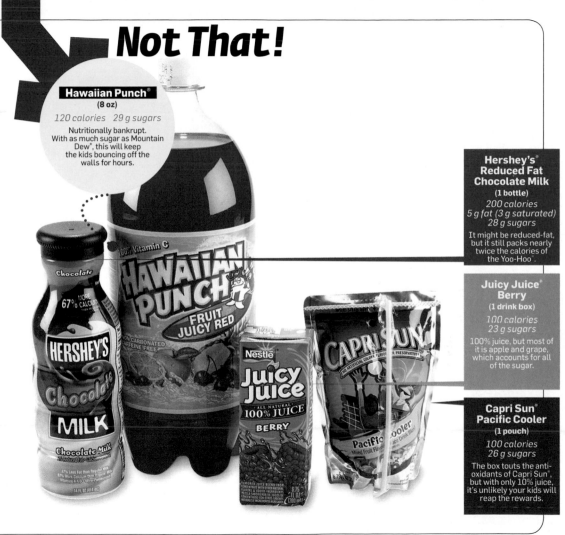

Hawaiian Punch®
(8 oz)

120 calories   29 g sugars

Nutritionally bankrupt.
With as much sugar as Mountain
Dew®, this will keep
the kids bouncing off the
walls for hours.

Hershey's®
Reduced Fat
Chocolate Milk
(1 bottle)

200 calories
5 g fat (3 g saturated)
28 g sugars

It might be reduced-fat,
but it still packs nearly
twice the calories of
the Yoo-Hoo®.

Juicy Juice®
Berry
(1 drink box)

100 calories
23 g sugars

100% juice, but most of
it is apple and grape,
which accounts for all
of the sugar.

Capri Sun®
Pacific Cooler
(1 pouch)

100 calories
26 g sugars

The box touts the anti-
oxidants of Capri Sun®,
but with only 10% juice,
it's unlikely your kids will
reap the rewards.

Smoothies & Shakes
Drink This

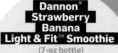

Dannon® Strawberry Banana Light & Fit™ Smoothie
(7-oz bottle)

70 calories
0 g fat   12 g sugars

Nonfat yogurt flavored with banana, strawberry, and apple puree. Exactly what you want to wake up to.

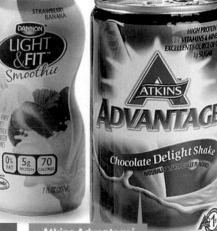

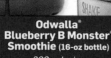

Odwalla® Blueberry B Monster® Smoothie (16-oz bottle)

280 calories
0 g fat
54 g sugars

720 percent of your daily allowance of thiamin, riboflavin, vitamin B_6, and vitamin B_{12}. Forget energy drinks: Thiamin converts sugar into energy, and riboflavin aids energy production.

Slim-Fast® High Protein Extra Creamy Vanilla Shake (11.5-oz can)

190 calories
5 g fat (2 g saturated)
13 g sugars

As a meal replacement, Slim-Fast® delivers 35 percent of your vitamin D and 100 percent of vitamins C and E. This high-protein variety halves the sugar and packs 15 grams of protein.

Atkins Advantage® Chocolate Delight Shake (11-oz can)

160 calories
9 g fat (2 g saturated)
1 g sugars

This shake packs 15 grams of protein and at least 30 percent of 14 different vitamins and minerals, including calcium, vitamin A, folate, riboflavin, and thiamin.

Not That!

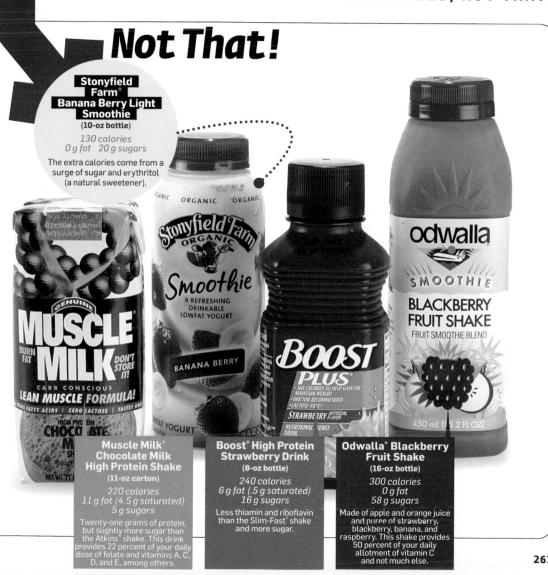

Stonyfield Farm® Banana Berry Light Smoothie
(10-oz bottle)

130 calories
0 g fat   20 g sugars

The extra calories come from a surge of sugar and erythritol (a natural sweetener).

Muscle Milk® Chocolate Milk High Protein Shake
(11-oz carton)

220 calories
11 g fat (4.5 g saturated)
5 g sugars

Twenty-one grams of protein, but slightly more sugar than the Atkins® shake. This drink provides 22 percent of your daily dose of folate and vitamins A, C, D, and E, among others.

Boost® High Protein Strawberry Drink
(8-oz bottle)

240 calories
6 g fat (.5 g saturated)
16 g sugars

Less thiamin and riboflavin than the Slim-Fast® shake and more sugar.

Odwalla® Blackberry Fruit Shake
(16-oz bottle)

300 calories
0 g fat
58 g sugars

Made of apple and orange juice and puree of strawberry, blackberry, banana, and raspberry. This shake provides 50 percent of your daily allotment of vitamin C and not much else.

Beer

Drink This

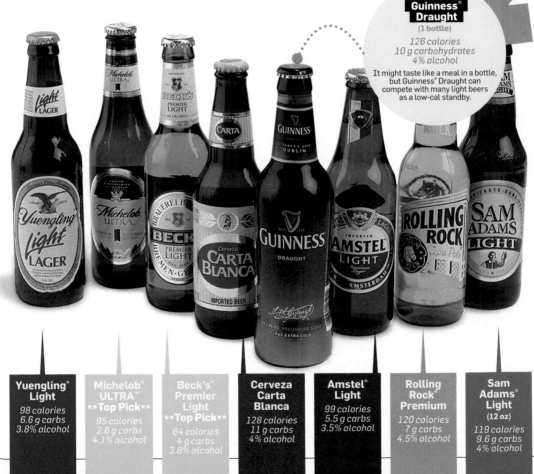

Guinness® Draught
(1 bottle)

126 calories
10 g carbohydrates
4% alcohol

It might taste like a meal in a bottle, but Guinness® Draught can compete with many light beers as a low-cal standby.

Yuengling® Light
98 calories
6.6 g carbs
3.8% alcohol

Michelob® ULTRA™
★★Top Pick★★
95 calories
2.6 g carbs
4.1% alcohol

Beck's® Premier Light
★★Top Pick★★
64 calories
4 g carbs
3.8% alcohol

Cerveza Carta Blanca
128 calories
11 g carbs
4% alcohol

Amstel® Light
99 calories
5.5 g carbs
3.5% alcohol

Rolling Rock® Premium
120 calories
7 g carbs
4.5% alcohol

Sam Adams® Light
(12 oz)
119 calories
9.6 g carbs
4% alcohol

Not That!

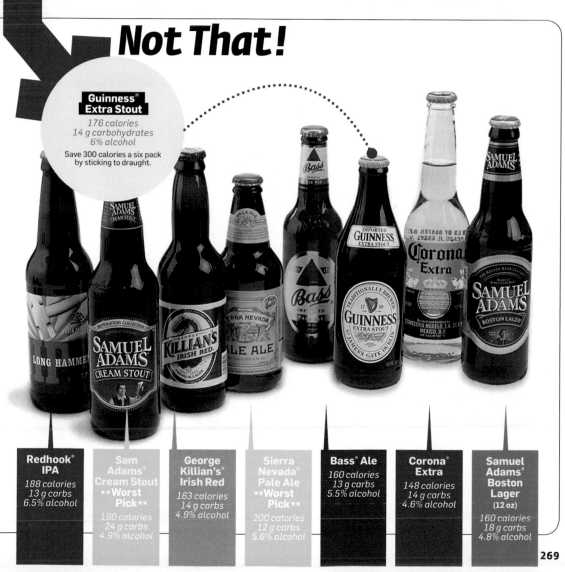

Guinness® Extra Stout

176 calories
14 g carbohydrates
6% alcohol

Save 300 calories a six pack by sticking to draught.

Redhook® IPA

188 calories
13 g carbs
6.5% alcohol

Sam Adams® Cream Stout ★★Worst Pick★★

190 calories
24 g carbs
4.9% alcohol

George Killian's® Irish Red

163 calories
14 g carbs
4.9% alcohol

Sierra Nevada® Pale Ale ★★Worst Pick★★

200 calories
12 g carbs
5.6% alcohol

Bass® Ale

160 calories
13 g carbs
5.5% alcohol

Corona® Extra

148 calories
14 g carbs
4.6% alcohol

Samuel Adams® Boston Lager (12 oz)

160 calories
18 g carbs
4.8% alcohol

269

Cocktails

Drink This

HANGOVER HELPERS

Gatorade

Alcohol inhibits secretion of the hormone vasopressin, bringing on dehydration, which exacerbates the symptoms of a hangover. Gatorade's 6 percent carbohydrate solution promotes rehydration better than mere water. It's also a great substitute because the extra salt helps your body absorb the fluid more quickly.

Drinking Only Light-colored Alcohol
(white wine, vodka, and gin)

Lighter drinks have fewer headache-inducing congeners than darker drinks, like red wine, beer, and dark liquors. It actually does work—but only if you're drinking in moderation.

Saltines
(10, to be exact, washed down with 24 oz water)

Salt helps you retain the fluid you lose over a night of drinking. With 32 milligrams of salt per cracker, this is a surefire way to keep from drying up.

The Mega-dinner

Food delays gastric emptying in the stomach—meaning alcohol stays there longer and is processed more slowly. Don't drink on an empty stomach: The longer alcohol stays in the stomach, the better your body breaks it down.

Bloody Mary
(8 oz)

140 calories 8 g carbs
150 mg sodium

This is one of the few mixed drinks that actually offers some nutritional benefits; made with low sodium V8®, this drink offers a healthy dose of vitamins C, A, and lycopene, the cancer-fighting antioxidant found in tomatoes.

Screwdriver
(6 oz)

130 calories
13 g carbs

Sure, the OJ gives the drink a surge of sugar, but unlike tonic and soft drink mixers, at least this one has some redeeming nutritional benefits.

Not That!

Margarita
(8 oz)

500 calories
32 g carbs

Pre-made margarita mixes, the standard in most bars and restaurants, are essentially high-fructose corn syrup laced with a trace amount of lime juice. Ask the bartender to make your margi' fresh, with only a small hit of sugar to balance the tartness of the lime.

8

The number of alcoholic drinks the average guy knocks back weekly. The average woman only has four.

Booze by the Numbers

Drink	Alcohol (g)	Calories
Red Wine (1 glass, 5 fl oz)	15.6	125
White Wine (1 glass, 5 fl oz)	15.1	121
Dessert Wine (1 glass, 3.5 fl oz)	15.8	165
Sake (1.5 fl.oz)	7	58
Rum 80 proof (1.5 fl oz)	14	97
Vodka 80 proof (1.5 fl oz)	14	97
Whiskey 86 proof (1.5 fl oz)	15.1	105
Gin 90 proof (1.5 fl oz)	15.9	110
Kahlua 53 proof (1.5 fl oz)	11.3	170
Whiskey Sour (1 cocktail)	15	169
Pina Colada (1 cocktail)	14	245
Tequila Sunrise (1 cocktail)	13.2	154

Gin and tonic
(6 oz)

140 calories
11 g carbs

There are 22 grams of sugar in an 8-ounce glass of tonic. Opt for sugar-free diet tonic, if available.

Rum and Diet Coke®
(6 oz)

110 calories
0 g carbs

Australian researchers found that mixing liquor with diet drinks can intensify the alcoholic effect by 50%.

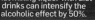

Chapter 7

WHAT TO EAT WHEN...

15 Foods that Cure

BEST BLOOD SUGAR STABILIZER: RASPBERRIES
Raspberries contain anthocyanins, which boost insulin production and lower blood sugar levels, providing a strong defense against diabetes.

BEST SKIN SAVER: CARROTS
National Cancer Institute researchers found that people with the highest intakes of carotenoids—pigments that occur naturally in carrots—were six times less likely to develop skin cancer than those with the lowest intakes.

BEST HEART PROTECTOR: SALMON
A diet of heart-healthy fats, like those found in salmon and olive oil, raises good HDL cholesterol levels. And salmon contains a huge dose of omega-3 fatty acids, which can ward off heart disease.

BEST BREAST CANCER BEATER: WHOLE-GRAIN CEREAL
Women getting at least 30 grams of fiber daily are half as likely to develop breast cancer, according to research. A bowl of Fiber One® with blueberries will get you halfway there.

BEST BONE PROTECTOR: SHRIMP
Shrimp is high in vitamin B12, which aids bone density and is crucial in the generation of new cells. It is also a good source of vitamin D, an essential ingredient for bone strength.

BEST COLON CANCER GUARD: GREEN OR WHITE TEA
Drinking just one cup of tea a day may cut your risk of colon cancer in half. Antioxidants in the tea, called catechins, inhibit the growth of cancer cells.

BEST VISION DEFENDER: SPINACH OR ROMAINE LETTUCE

The National Institutes of Health found that people who consume the most lutein—found in leafy greens—are 43 percent less likely to develop macular degeneration.

BEST ANTI-AGING ELIXIR: RED WINE

Oxidative stress plays a major role in aging, and an antioxidant in red wine called resveratrol may help extend life by neutralizing disease-causing free radicals. Pop a Pinot Noir: It packs the most resveratrol per glass.

BEST LUNG CANCER FIGHTER: GRAPEFRUIT

A grapefruit a day can reduce your risk of developing lung cancer by up to 50 percent. Grapefruit contains naringin, which may help lower levels of cancer-causing enzymes.

BEST PROSTATE PROTECTOR: GARLIC

Compounds in garlic have been shown to reduce risk of prostate cancer by up to 50 percent.

BEST CAVITY KILLER: MONTEREY JACK CHEESE

Researchers found that eating less than a quarter ounce of Jack, Cheddar, Gouda, or mozzarella cheese will boost pH levels to protect your pearly whites from cavities.

BEST HAIR REJUVENATOR: BEEF

Iron in the meat stimulates hair turnover and replenishment. Beef is also rich in zinc, which helps guard against hair loss.

BEST CHOLESTEROL REDUCER: OLIVE OIL

Antioxidants found in olives have been shown both to raise HDL (good) cholesterol and lower LDL (bad) cholesterol, making olive oil a doubly potent protector against cardiovascular disease.

BEST BLOOD PRESSURE REDUCER: BAKED POTATO

Increasing the amount of potassium in your diet (a baked potato will boost your intake by about 400 mg, but be sure to eat the skin!) will significantly lower your blood pressure.

BEST BRAIN BOOSTER: COFFEE

Beyond boosting alertness for up to 90 minutes, that morning cup is the number-one source of antioxidants in the American diet, and can help decrease your risk of developing Alzheimer's disease by as much as 60 percent.

When You're Stressed

MODERN LIFE IS A BIG, boiling cauldron of anxiety stew, and we get a heaping helping every day. Whether you're talking to your boss about a promotion, talking to your spouse about the credit card bills, or talking to your kids about a streak of bad behavior, there's always a stress-soaked moment around the corner. So calm yourself quick with these natural nerve-settlers.

Did You Know?
Researchers at the University of Bristol in England discovered that when stressed-out men consumed caffeine by themselves, they remained nervous and jittery. But when anxious men caffeine-loaded as part of a group, their feelings of stress subsided.

Eat This **1 CUP OF LOW-FAT YOGURT or 2 TBSP OF MIXED NUTS**
Scientists in Slovakia gave people 3 grams each of two amino acids—lysine and arginine—or a placebo and asked them to deliver a speech. Blood measurements of stress hormones revealed that the amino acid—fortified guys were half as anxious during and after the speech as those who took the placebo. Yogurt is one of the best food sources of lysine; nuts pack tons of arginine.

RED BELL PEPPERS
Researchers at the University of Alabama fed rats 200 milligrams of vitamin C twice a day and found that it nearly stopped the secretion of stress hormones. Add half a sliced red bell pepper to a salad or sandwich; calorie for calorie, no single food gives you more vitamin C.

A CUP OF PEPPERMINT TEA
The scent of peppermint helps you focus and boosts performance, according to researchers. In another study, they found that peppermint makes drivers more alert and less anxious.

A HANDFUL OF SESAME SEEDS
Stress hormones can deplete your body's supply of magnesium, reducing your stress-coping abilities and increasing your risk of developing high blood pressure. Sesame seeds are packed with this essential mineral.

Not That! **A CAN OF SODA**
A study from the American Journal of Public Health found that people who drink 2½ cans of soda daily are three times more likely to be depressed and anxious, compared with those who drink fewer.

When You're Sad

WATCH ENOUGH TV ADVERTISING and you begin to think the only answer to a bad mood is a bottle of pills. Wrong! Your next meal can have as dramatic an impact on your mood as your next prescription refill. So the next time you have a gnawing feeling that something's amiss, try gnawing on one of these.

Eat This

AN ARUGULA or SPINACH SALAD

Leafy greens—arugula, chard, spinach—are rich sources of B vitamins, which are part of the assembly line that manufactures feel-good hormones such as serotonin, dopamine, and norepinephrine. In fact, according to a study published in the *Journal of Neuroscience Nursing*, a lack of B6 can cause nervousness, irritability, and even depression.

TUNA SASHIMI or GRILLED SALMON

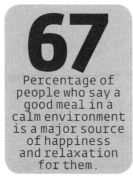

67

Percentage of people who say a good meal in a calm environment is a major source of happiness and relaxation for them.

A study in Finland found that people who eat more fish are 31 percent less likely to suffer from depression. And skip sweet, simple carbs (like the rice with your sushi)—the inevitable sugar crash can deepen depression.

1 TBSP OF GROUND FLAXSEED DAILY

Flax is the best source of alpha-linoleic acid, or ALA—a healthy fat that improves the workings of the cerebral cortex, the area of the brain that processes sensory information, including that of pleasure. To meet your quota, sprinkle it on salads or mix it to in a smoothie or shake.

Not That!

WHITE CHOCOLATE

White chocolate isn't technically chocolate, since it contains no cocoa solids. That means it also lacks the ability to stimulate the euphoria-inducing chemicals that real chocolate does, especially serotonin. If you're going to grab some chocolate, darker is better; more cacao means more happy chemicals and less sugar, which will eventually pull you down.

Did You Know?

People who frequently eat high-fiber foods have a more positive outlook on life and are less likely to have symptoms of depression than people who eat less fiber, according to a new UK study.

When You're Feeling Fat

WHETHER YOU'RE TRYING to revert to prom-era size for your high school reunion or recovering from a season of holiday bingeing, you want to get rid of the extra pounds—and that sluggish feeling—in a hurry. So don't tailor your clothes—tailor your meals.

Eat This

GRILLED CHICKEN BREAST The protein in lean meat and poultry fills you up and speeds metabolism, which cuts your cravings while easing off the pounds. High-protein diets also help to build muscle and attack extra belly fat.

46

Percentage by which eating one grapefruit a day reduces narrowing of your arteries. The one-a-day grapefruit method can also lower your bad-cholesterol level by more than 10 percent and drop your blood pressure 5 points.

GRAPEFRUIT A grapefruit a day in addition to your regular meals can speed weight loss. The fruit's acidity slows digestion, helping you feel full longer. And the vitamin C—packed grapefruit works to lower cholesterol and decrease risk of stroke, heart disease, and some types of cancer.

A SMALL SCOOP OF TUNA SALAD (SANS BREAD) A study at the University of Oxford in England found that eating salmon and tuna can speed up the movement of food from your stomach to your intestines, which leaves your stomach calmer and quells bloating. Credit the omega-3 fatty acids found in the fish, which stimulate hormones that regulate food intake, body weight, and metabolism.

Not That!

CANNED SOUP AND SALTY SNACKS Sodium binges can lead to water retention, which makes your stomach feel like a beach ball. Avoid inflation by skipping salty foods like salted nuts and potato chips, and resist your cravings for Chinese takeout and Mexican food, two of the most salt-laden cuisines.

Did You Know?
Losing weight could be as easy as kicking your soda dependency. Replacing a 20-ounce soft drink with water will save you about 200 calories a day—that's 21 pounds a year!

When You're Low on Energy

IN SPANISH CULTURE, the siesta is a midday nap that replenishes the body's energy and prepares it for an evening of hard work and hard partying. Sadly, explaining a 3 p.m. snooze in such terms to your boss probably won't go very far. Instead, use this arsenal of foods to power through the midday slump.

Eat This

A HANDFUL OF TRAIL MIX
Raisins provide potassium, which your body uses to convert sugar into energy. Nuts stock your body with magnesium, which is important in metabolism, nerve function, and muscle function. (When magnesium levels are low, your body produces more lactic acid—the same a fatigue-inducing substance that you feel at the end of a long workout.)

A BOWL OF CEREAL
Cereal is an excellent source of thiamin and riboflavin. Both vitamins help your body use energy efficiently, so you won't be nodding off mid-PowerPoint.

HIGH-PROTEIN SALAD WITH VINAIGRETTE
The oil in the dressing will help slow down digestion of protein and carbs in the salad, stabilizing blood-sugar levels and keeping energy levels high. Build your salad on a bed of romaine and spinach for an added boost in riboflavin, and add chicken and a hard-boiled egg for energizing protein.

Not That!

ESPRESSO-BASED DRINKS
Sure, the caffeine will perk you up, but with anywhere from 16 grams (latte) to 59 grams (white chocolate mocha) of sugar in your Starbucks drink of choice, the spike in blood sugar will ultimately send you crashing. Stick to brewed coffee.

PANCAKES AND BAGELS
MIT researchers analyzed blood samples from a group of people who had eaten either a high-protein or a high-carbohydrate breakfast. Two hours after eating, the carb eaters had tryptophan levels four times higher than those of the people who had eaten protein. The higher your tryptophan level, the more likely you are to feel tired and sluggish.

Did You Know?
Harvard researchers found that people who replaced 127 calories of carbohydrates—that's about 14 Baked Lay's® potato chips—with 1 ounce of nuts decreased their risk of heart disease by 30 percent.

When You Need a Brain Boost

WHETHER YOU'RE trying to negotiate a mortgage, map a route to the Grand Canyon, or just help Junior with his calculus homework, you have to muster your smarts when the pressure's on. Stock up on these foods to slow cognitive decline, improve your memory, and protect your mental sharpness into old age.

Eat This

BLUEBERRIES

Antioxidants in blueberries help protect the brain from free-radical damage, which could decrease your risk of Alzheimer's and Parkinson's diseases, and improve cognitive processing. Wild blueberries, if you can find them, have even more brain-boosting antioxidants than the cultivated variety.

COFFEE

Fresh-brewed joe is the ultimate brain fuel. Caffeine has been shown to retard the aging process and enhance short-term memory performance. In one study, British researchers found that people consuming the caffeine equivalent of one cup of coffee experienced improved attention and problem-solving skills.

SALMON OR MACKEREL

The omega-3 fatty acids found in fish are one of the primary building blocks of brain tissue, so they're essential to boosting brain power. Salmon is also rich in niacin, which wards off Alzheimer's disease and slows the rate of cognitive decline.

Not That!

ICE CREAM

Sugary foods incite sudden surges of glucose that, in the long term, cause sugar highs and lows, leading to a lack of concentration. And foods high in saturated fat can clog blood vessels and prevent the flow of nutrients and blood to the brain.

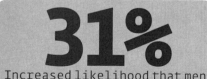

31%

Increased likelihood that men and women who eat fish less than once a week will be depressed, compared to those who eat fish twice a week.

Did You Know?
Women are less prone to memory loss than are men. The hormone progesterone protects neurotransmitters in the female brain.

When You Want to Increase Metabolism

WHO DOESN'T WANT a little help from this natural fat-burning engine? These foods will get the pistons pumping.

Eat This

GREEN TEA

Catechins, the powerful antioxidants found in green tea, are known to increase metabolism. A study by Japanese researchers found that participants who consumed 690 milligrams of catechins from green tea daily had significantly lower body mass indexes and smaller waist measurements than those in a control group.

STEAK & EGGS

A British study found that participants who increased the percentage of protein-based calories in their diets burned 71 more calories a day (that's 7.4 pounds a year). Jump-start your metabolism as soon as you wake up with a protein-rich breakfast of scrambled eggs and end your day with 4-6 ounces of high-quality protein like lean beef, chicken, or fish.

METABOLIC MATH

Your metabolism—the rate at which your body burns calories—experiences a drastic dip from your teen years into your 20s and 30s. But you can help counteract the decline: Physical activity makes up 15 to 30 percent of the average person's metabolism.

Did You Know?

Skipping meals lets your body's calorie-burning furnace go cold. Spread out snacks throughout the day. Try a cup of yogurt with fresh fruit or almonds at 10:30 a.m., and a hard-boiled egg or hummus with vegetables around 3 p.m.

SECRET WEAPON

YERBA MATE

This Argentinean plant used to make tea has been shown to contain up to 90 percent more metabolism-boosting catechins than green tea. In fact, its metabolic powers are so revered that many weight loss pills list mate on their ingredient lists. Score bottles of yerba mate at your local Whole Foods, or go online to guayaki.com and order leaves to brew your own fat-burning formula.

When You Need to Get Some Sleep

NOTHING MAKES IT HARDER to fall asleep than knowing how important it is to fall asleep. So when the pressure's on, try chowing on one of these snacks before bedtime to ensure some serious shut-eye.

Eat This

NONFAT POPCORN
Pop a bag half an hour before bedtime: The carbs will induce your body to create serotonin, a neurochemical that makes you feel relaxed. Skip the butter—fat will slow the process of boosting serotonin levels.

OATMEAL WITH SLICED BANANA AND WALNUTS
Sleep is inspired by the hormone melatonin, but stress or excitement can disrupt melatonin's release. Bring your brain back down to earth by whipping up a bowl of instant oatmeal and topping it with a sliced banana and crushed walnuts, both rich in melatonin.

A HANDFUL OF SESAME SEEDS
Sesame seeds are one of the best natural sources of tryptophan, the sleep-inducing amino acid responsible for all of those post-Thanksgiving turkey comas.

Not That!

A GLASS OF WARM MILK
Forget what your mom told you: This popular remedy for sleeplessness could be making matters worse. The protein in milk boosts alertness. Plus, unless it's skim, the fat in milk slows down digestion and makes sleep more fitful.

Did You Know?
Harvard scientists found that people who slept for 5 hours or less a night were 32 percent more likely to pack on major extra pounds (33 pounds) than those who dozed a full 7 hours.

9
Number of hours that even small amounts of caffeine can disrupt sleep

---

SECRET WEAPON

CHERRY JUICE
Researchers at the University of Texas found that tart cherries are one of the best natural sources of melatonin. You can keep the pits off the sheets by drinking juices made with cherry concentrate; they have 10 times the melatonin content of the fruit. Try Knudsen® Just Black Cherry™, with 100% cherry juice and no added sugar.

When You Need to Wake Up and Go

SKIP BREAKFAST and you'll drag all day—and even put on pounds. But put the right stuff on your plate—or in your bowl—and you'll burn fat and have enough energy to breeze through the morning.

Eat This

EGGS AND WHOLE WHEAT TOAST

Eggs are a great source of protein, and having them for breakfast sets you up for a perfect day of eating. Saint Louis University researchers found that people who eat eggs for breakfast consume 264 fewer calories the rest of the day than those who eat bagels and cream cheese.

COTTAGE CHEESE TOPPED WITH BERRIES

If you want that energy to last until lunch, leggo the Eggo and the Aunt Jemima. You need a breakfast that will produce slow and steady levels of blood sugar, not a sudden spike. Try a combination of protein and fiber-rich carbs, such as cottage cheese topped with berries, or two scrambled eggs stuffed into a whole wheat pita.

POST® ORIGINAL SHREDDED WHEAT

Breakfast cereals should have at least 5 grams of fiber, and no more than 5 grams of sugar per serving. The fiber will help keep your belly full and your blood sugar levels stable. Too boring for you? Add some sliced strawberries, a few tablespoons of raisins or a handful of blueberries.

Not That!

BAGEL AND CREAM CHEESE

At 500 calories and 20 grams of fat, this classic is one of the worst ways to start your day. 60 grams of fast-burning carbohydrates will cause a dip in energy and a spike in hunger, long before lunchtime. The same goes for croissants, danish, donuts, and pancakes.

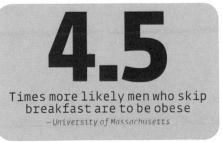

4.5

Times more likely men who skip breakfast are to be obese
—University of Massachusetts

Did You Know?

Waiting more than 90 minutes after waking to eat breakfast may increase your chances of obesity by nealy 50 percent.

When You're Hung Over

IT WAS SUPPOSED TO BE a few quick ones at Happy Hour, but now you're facing Very Unhappy Morning, and you've still got to plow through the day. After a boozy night out, these remedies will soothe your dragging body.

Eat This

ORANGE JUICE
For last call, order a double virgin screwdriver. Fructose, one of the sugars in orange juice, can speed the metabolism of alcohol by as much as 25 percent. Vitamin C also helps combat binge-related cell damage.

COLD WATER OR GATORADE®
These no-brainers are the best relievers of a hangover. They replace the fluid lost through urine and sweat, dilute the acid in your irritated stomach, and lower body temperature. Every ounce of alcohol needs to be replaced by 18 ounces of water. A sports drink is even better, as it replaces electrolytes.

50
Percent larger a self-poured cocktail is than a standard drink, according to researchers at the Alcohol Research Group in California.

TOAST WITH PRESERVES OR BERRIES
These antioxidant-packed fruits counter low blood sugar, and the toast relieves nausea. As with orange juice, the fructose in berries can help you recover by speeding the rate at which your body metabolizes last night's booze.

Not That!

WHISKEY AND DIET COKE®
Skip this classic and you may sidestep the hangover entirely. An Australian study found that mixing liquor with a diet drink nearly doubles your blood alcohol content. And darker-colored alcohols like whiskey, brandies, and red wine are more likely to cause a hangover than lighter-colored alcohols, like gin and vodka. This is because darker liquors contain more congeners—impurities that are the by-products of fermentation and aging—for your body to process.

Did You Know?
The lowest-calorie drink options are vodka with club soda or a scotch and water—each has about 100 calories, as does a light beer or a glass of white wine. But happy hour is also prone to boosting your appetite, so beware of the munchies.

When You're Under the Weather

THE FIRST LINE OF DEFENSE in the war on your well-being isn't found in the pharmacy—it's in the aisles of the supermarket. Warm up your cold, send the flu flying, and bolster your immune system with these foods.

Eat This

GINSENG TEA, HOT OR ICED

In a Canadian study, people who took 400 milligrams of ginseng a day had 25 percent fewer colds than those popping a placebo. Ginseng helps kill invading viruses by increasing the body's production of key immune cells.

GREEN TEA

EGCG, a chemical compound that is potent in green tea, has been shown to stop the adenovirus (one of the bugs responsible for colds) from replicating. Start pumping green tea into your system at the first sign of a cold and you should be able to stave off worse symptoms. The best brand to brew? Go with Tetley®; it was the most effective brand in studies.

ORANGES

The zinc and vitamin C in oranges won't prevent the onslaught of a cold, but it might decrease the severity and duration of your symptoms. One orange provides more than 100 percent of your daily recommended intake of vitamin C.

OLIVE OIL AND AVOCADOS

Foods rich in healthy fats, such as olive oil and avocados, help reduce inflammation, a catalyst for migraines. One study found that the anti-inflammatory compound in olive oil suppresses the same pain pathway as ibuprofen.

Not That!

CAFFEINATED BEVERAGES AND ENERGY DRINKS

Excessive caffeine screws with your sleep schedule and suppresses functions of key immune agents. And insufficient sleep opens the door to colds, upper respiratory infections, and other ills. What's more, caffeine can dehydrate you, and hydration is vital during illness: Fluids not only transport nutrients to the illness site, but also dispose of toxins.

Did You Know?
Hang with friends to bolster your disease-fighting power: Isolation can cause stress and sap your immune system.

When You Want to Get "In the Mood"

THE IDEA OF AN APHRODISIAC has been around since early man pulled the first oyster from the ocean and decided it reminded him of early woman. But not all passion foods are quite so expensive—and they don't need to be eaten raw. Unleash these mood foods to boost arousal and sexual stamina.

Eat This

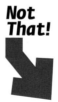

DARK CHOCOLATE

The cocoa in chocolate contains methylxanthines, stimulants that increase your body's sensitivity. Chocolate also contains phenylethylamine, a chemical that can give you a slight natural high. And Italian researchers found that women who often eat chocolate have a higher sex drive than those who don't. Make sure your chocolate has at least 60 percent cacao.

SIX-OUNCE SIRLOIN STEAK

Protein has been shown to naturally boost levels of dopamine and norepinephrine, two chemicals in the brain that heighten sensitivity during sex. Your steak is also packed with zinc—a mineral that

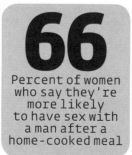

66
Percent of women who say they're more likely to have sex with a man after a home-cooked meal

boosts libido by reducing production of a hormone called prolactin, which may interfere with arousal.

VANILLA ICE CREAM

Ice cream has high levels of calcium and phosphorus, two minerals that build your muscles' energy reserves and boost your libido. All that calcium (200 milligrams in the typical bowl) can also make your orgasms more powerful, since the muscles that control ejaculation and orgasm need calcium in order to spasm and contract properly.

Not That!

A BOTTLE OF WINE

While a drink or two can increase arousal signals between your brain and your genitals, more than a few drinks will actually depress your nervous system, making it harder for men to maintain an erection. Split a bottle with your partner, but stop there.

Did You Know?

Studies show both sexes experience a surge of libido-boosting testosterone 30 minutes after a workout.

When You Want a Baby

IT'S ONE OF LIFE'S GREAT IRONIES that couples who spend their teens and 20s trying to avoid getting pregnant often find themselves in their 30s and 40s doing just the opposite. While the miracle of conception depends on many factors, you can tweak the odds in your favor through a careful diet.

Eat This

BRAZIL NUTS
Cigarette smoke, air pollution, and other toxins in the air can damage sperm, altering the DNA inside the cells and possibly increasing your child's risk of birth defects. Your best bet? Call in the Brazilians. Brazil nuts are a top source of selenium, a mineral that boosts sperm health while also helping the little buggers swim faster.

LIVER
It might not sound sexy, but ounce for ounce there are few better sources of fertility-boosting vitamin A than liver. Studies show that men who get plenty of A each day have higher sperm counts and perform better sexually than men who don't. Can't stomach the liver? Try a salad made with red leaf lettuce and shredded carrots.

FROZEN PEACHES
University of Texas researchers found that men who consumed at least 200 milligrams of vitamin C a day had higher sperm counts than men who took in less. Vitamin C also keeps sperm from clumping, meaning they'll have a better chance of finding their target. Keep a bag of frozen peach slices—they have more C than fresh ones do—in your freezer to dump in smoothies or add to your morning cereal. A single cup of the fruit has more than twice your daily vitamin C requirement.

Not That!

DONUTS AND FRIES
Researchers from Harvard found that women who took in 2 percent of their calories from trans fats had a 70 percent greater risk of infertility than those who consumed no trans fats at all. Avoid fast food and chain restaurants that still fry in trans fat–laden oil, and skip packaged foods like chips and cookies with partially hydrogenated oils on the ingredient list.

Did You Know?
According to the Mayo Clinic, spending more than 30 minutes in a bath or hot tub above 102°F may significantly lower sperm count.

When You Want to Look and Feel Younger

WHETHER TO AVOID WRINKLES, protect your ticker, or keep your mind sharp, proper eating is the only real fountain of youth.

Eat This

SUNFLOWER SEEDS

These tiny wonders have the highest natural vitamin E content of any food around, and no antioxidant is better at fighting off the aging effects of free radicals. Other great sources of vitamin E include Swiss chard, Total® Cereal and Propel® Fitness Water.

SPINACH AND BEANS

Researchers studied the diets of 400 elderly men and women, and found that those who ate the most leafy green vegetables and beans had the fewest wrinkles. The reason? Spinach and beans are full of compounds that help prevent and repair wear and tear on your skin cells as you get older.

RED WINE AND GRAPE JUICE

Besides providing protection from heart attack and stroke, the antioxidants called polyphenols found in grapes can also help keep middle-aged skin from sagging.

SWEET POTATOES

Overexposure to the sun is one of the primary reasons men age prematurely. But European researchers recently found that pigments from beta carotene-rich foods like sweet potatoes and carrots can build up in your skin, helping to prevent damage from ultraviolet rays.

COFFEE

One of nature's most potent elixirs, coffee has been shown in numerous studies to retard the aging process, fight off Alzheimer's disease, and enhance short-term memory.

Did You Know?

Dutch researchers found that people who took 800 mcg of folic acid every day—the amount in a serving of Total Whole Grain cereal—exhibited memories that were 5 to 8 years younger than those who didn't.

1

Rank of coffee among the highest sources of antioxidants in the American diet. Antioxidants are critical in picking off free radicals that cause cancer.

—*University of Scranton*

When You Want the Most from Your Workout

THE RIGHT POST-WORKOUT MEALS help build lean muscle, repair your body, and ensure gains long after you've done your last rep.

Eat This

PB & J OR PASTA

The perfect post-weight training repast has about 400 calories, with 20 to 30 grams of protein (to build new muscle) and 50 to 65 grams of carbohydrates (to repair old muscle). Peanut butter and jelly sandwiches or a small bowl of pasta with meat sauce fit that formula.

PORK TENDERLOIN

Lean meats are a great low-calorie source of protein, and scientists at McMaster University in Hamilton, Ontario, found that eating more protein may reduce the fat around your midsection. People who ate 20 more grams of protein every day than the group average had 6 percent lower waist-to-hip ratios.

PINEAPPLE AND PAPAYA

Both of these tropical fruits are loaded with bromelain and papain, enzymes that not only help break down proteins for digestion, but also have anti-inflammatory properties to speed up your post-workout recovery.

MILK

The best sports drink may come from a cow. British researchers found that milk does a better job than water or sports drinks at rehydrating the body after exercise. Why? Because milk has more electrolytes and potassium.

COFFEE

University of Georgia scientists revealed that taking a caffeine supplement (equal to 2 cups of coffee) after exercise reduces muscle soreness more than pain relievers can. Caffeine blocks a chemical that activates pain receptors.

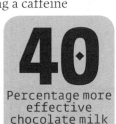

40

Percentage more effective chocolate milk is at repairing muscles after a workout than plain milk.
—University of Washington

Did You Know?

After exercise, munch immediately—ideally, within 30 minutes of working out—so your body doesn't begin breaking down muscle tissue to replenish itself.

289

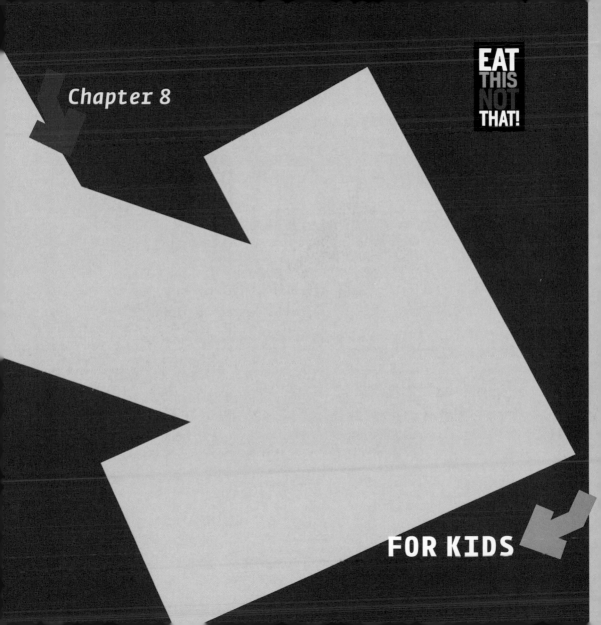

Chapter 8

EAT
THIS
NOT
THAT!

FOR KIDS

Feeding the Future

Just as the waistline of the average adult American is expanding at a belt-breaking rate, so too are those of this country's youth. It doesn't take a nutritionist to see that almost overnight we've gone from Generation X to Generation XXL. Recent research shows that kids today consume 180 calories more per day compared to kids in 1989, and all of those extra calories translate into some pretty staggering health consequences: 45 percent of this country's youth are overweight or obese, and the number of children burdened with diabetes has nearly quadrupled in the past thirty years.

Only 2 percent—that's right, 2 percent—of children between the ages of 2 and 19 are fulfilling their five main recommendations for a healthy diet laid out in the USDA's Food Guide Pyramid. That means a serious dearth of whole grains, fruit, vegetables, dairy, and lean proteins and an excess of sugar-filled packaged foods. In fact, a study of 4,000 children of that same age group showed that the overwhelming bulk of their nutrients come from cereals and fruit drinks. If kids are relying on Frosted Flakes® and Hawaiian Punch® for nutrition, we know there's a problem.

Legislation is in effect across the country to try to control the flow of food into our schools. But you can't afford to wait for a group of strangers in suits to pass laws that tell your kids how to eat. According to a report issued by researchers at Baylor College of Medicine, a student who enters high school overweight has only a slight chance of reaching a normal weight by adulthood. High school freshmen at healthy weights, on the other hand, are four times as likely to stay slim as adults.

We all need help with our diets, especially kids. Use the guidelines and tips below to lay the foundation for a life of healthy eating.

DAILY NEEDS*

2 TO 3 YEARS OLD: (Boys and girls) *1,200 calories*	4 TO 8 YEARS OLD:		9 TO 13 YEARS OLD:	
	Girls *1,500 calories*	Boys *1,700 calories*	Girls *1,900 calories*	Boys *2,100 calories*
1 cup of fruits	1.5 cups fruits	1.5 cups fruits	2 cups fruits	2 cups fruits
1.4 cups of vegetables	2 cups vegetables	2.5 cups vegetables	2.5 cups vegetables	3 cups vegetables
4 oz whole grains	5 oz grains	5.5 oz grains	6 oz grains	6.5 oz grains
3 oz meat and beans	5 oz meat and beans	5 oz meat and beans	5.5 oz meat and beans	6.5 oz meat and beans
2 cups milk	2.5 cups milk	3 cups milk	3 cups milk	3 cups milk
4 tsp oils	4 tsp oils	5 tsp oils	5 tsp oils	6 tsp oils

*According to the USDA; ±300 calories and ±1 serving, depending on daily physical activity

Eat This

CALCIUM: Only 30 percent of children consume the recommended number of servings of milk each day. Avoid brittle bones by pouring them a glass of calcium-enhanced orange juice for breakfast, or by making a cup of low-fat, low-sugar yogurt or string cheese part of their daily snack routine.
FIBER: Besides keeping our bellies feeling full, fiber plays a vital role in regulating blood sugar levels, which makes it a potent weapon against one of the biggest health threats facing kids today: type II diabetes. The American Health Foundation recommends that a child's fiber intake be equivalent to his or her age plus 5 grams a day. Start their days with a bowl of cereal with at least 5 grams of fiber per serving and send them off to school with a high-fiber fruit like raspberries, a banana, or a sliced apple.
VITAMIN A: Only about one-third of males and females 12 to 19 years old consume the recommended daily amount of vitamin A. Vitamin A is essential in developing and strengthening our immune systems, improving vision, and aiding in healthy cell growth. Try pairing baby carrots with peanut butter for an afternoon snack.
IRON: According to a survey by the USDA, 60 percent of children 5 years and younger, 60 percent of females 6 to 11 years old, and only 28 percent of females 12 to 19 years old consume

100 percent or more of the recommended daily allowance for iron. Celery sticks, sliced tomatoes, and baked sweet potatoes are all solid sources of iron.

VITAMIN C: Only one in five children consume the recommended 5 servings of fruits and vegetables a day and one-quarter of all vegetables that are consumed are French fries. Opt for whole fruit—oranges, watermelon, pineapple—over juice whenever possible and make sure dinner always comes accompanied with at least one serving of colorful vegetables like peppers, asparagus, or carrots.

5 Hidden Dangers for Kids

These five foods find their way into the daily diet of most American kids, but they could be doing more harm than good.

● **CEREAL:** The vast majority of cereals that kids beg for are loaded with added sugars; a bowl of Trix or Lucky Charms® has more sugar than most ice cream bars. Watch out for sneaky serving sizes, too: Pressured by the USDA and concerned parents across the country to improve the nutritional content of cereals marketed to children, many cereal manufacturers simply shrank the serving sizes on their nutrition labels rather than cleaning up their act.

● **JUICE:** Most of the individually packaged "juices" like Capri Sun® and Sunny Delight® are merely glorified sugar water, with token amounts of real fruit juice. Even 100% juice drinks don't always deliver the best nutrition; whenever possible, avoid giving the little ones grape and apple juice, which have very high rates of naturally occurring sugars. Instead, opt for orange, cranberry, or even grapefruit juice.

● **LUNCH SNACKS:** "Fruit" snacks might as well be called gummy bears, and most granola bars, bound together by high-fructose corn syrup, are only a small step up from candy bars. Before making a snack a permanent fixture in their lunch boxes, read the label and make sure the food is free of or very low in high-fructose corn syrup and has less than 10 grams of sugar. Send them off instead with high-protein, low-sugar snacks like string cheese, almonds, or peanut butter and crackers.

● **BREAD:** White bread, specifically. Supermarket white breads are loaded with refined white flour and high-fructose corn syrup (yes, they even sweeten our breads now), both of which are known to spike blood sugar and set the little ones up for a serious carb crash. Start them early on whole grain breads (with at least 3 g of fiber a slice) and they'll be believers for life.

● **VEGETABLES:** Not vegetables, but what you let your kids put on them. Pass them the bottle of Cheez Whiz® or ranch dressing every time you steam a head of broccoli and it will be a decade before they learn to get down a floret without a cloak of saturated fat.

Not That!

FAT: The USDA and National Cholesterol Education Program recommend reducing fat intake to an average of 30 percent of calories or less for children over 2 years old.

SATURATED FAT: Saturated fat intake should be an average of less than 10 percent of calories for those over 2 years old, according to the USDA.

SUGARS: A child's diet should have 35 percent or less of its total calories from sugars, excluding sugars occurring naturally in fruits and vegetables, according to the Center for Science in the Public Interest. Soft drink consumption has doubled over the last 30 years. (Teenage boys consume twice the recommended amount of sugar each day, almost one-half of which comes from soft drinks; teenage girls fare even worse.) Each daily serving of sugar-sweetened soda increases a child's risk for obesity by 60 percent.

TO SPUR GROWTH
Eat This

WHOLE GRAIN CEREAL WITH VITAMIN D MILK: The calcium and vitamin D found in a bowl of cereal builds strong bones, which are essential for childhood development. According to study in the Journal of the American Dietetic Association, fortified foods such as cereal are a major source of essential nutrients like vitamin A, iron, and folate in toddlers, and this contribution increases as children age. Opt for milk instead of juice for lunch and dinner: not only does it aid bone growth, low-fat milk also has been shown to lower kids' risk of developing insulin resistance, which can lead to type 2 diabetes.

Not That!

SODA: Soda and sweetened fruit juices are likely to make your kids grow fatter, not taller. In a study at Cornell University, children who drank more than 16 ounces of sweetened drinks like juice or soda each day gained an average of $2\frac{1}{2}$ pounds over 2 months. And kids who are overweight are 9 percent more likely to suffer a bone fracture at some point during childhood or adolescence than fit kids. Overweight kids are also more likely to suffer from joint, bone, or muscle pain later in life.

TO FEED A DEVELOPING BRAIN:
Eat This

ROAST BEEF: Rotate roast beef sandwiches into your child's lunch schedule. Lean meat is a good source of iron and B vitamins, both nutrients that fuel the brain. Vitamin B6 is directly involved in the synthesis of neurotransmitters, and eating foods rich in B vitamins can soothe anxiety. During development, iron is crucial in fetal development, and iron deficiency has been linked with lower IQ, attention-deficit disorder, and hyperactivity disorder in children.

BREAKFAST: Make sure not to rush out without breakfast! According to a study at Harvard University, students who started eating breakfast were more likely to consume the daily recommended allowance for vitamins and minerals and to show improvements in academic performance (including higher math scores) and behavior.

Not That!

NON-ORGANIC PRODUCE AND JUICES: According to researchers from the University of Washington, kids who eat conventional produce have pesticide metabolite levels that are up to six times greater than those who eat organic foods. Research suggests that these metabolites can lead to problems in neurological functioning, neurological development, and growth in children.

TO PROMOTE BETTER BEHAVIOR:

Eat This

LEGUMES, FRUITS, VEGETABLES: High-sugar or carb-loaded kid staples like fruit snacks, granola bars, and white bread provide a temporary euphoric buzz, followed by an afternoon crash as your kid's blood sugar—and mood—plummet. Instead, opt for snacks with a low glycemic index, meaning they cause a smaller disturbance in blood sugar levels for no cranky withdrawal stage. Foods like vegetables, fruits, beans, and peanuts provide kids with an energy boost while keeping insulin levels stable.

MULTIVITAMINS: Another reason for Junior to take his vitamins. Studies have shown that school-age children with behavioral problems experience significant improvements in their classroom behavior after adding a multivitamin to their diets.

Not That!

HIGHLY PROCESSED FOODS, LIKE FROZEN WAFFLES, OR FOODS CONTAINING ARTIFICIAL COLORS AND PRESERVATIVES, LIKE DORITOS® OR CANDY: They might beg for junk food when they're cranky, but they'll only make your kid's mood worse.

Apart from the obvious cache of carbs and sugar, highly processed foods may have another adverse effect on kids' moods: British researchers found that artificial food colorings and preservatives in their diets caused an increase in hyperactive behavior in 3-year-olds. (Likewise, a withdrawal of such preservatives caused a significant reduction in hyperactivity.) An Australian study found that foods with synthetic food coloring such as tartrazine (Yellow 5—the kind found in Doritos®) was linked with irritability, restlessness, and sleep disturbance in children.

TO BOOST ENERGY:
Eat This
ALL-NATURAL PEANUT BUTTER ON WHOLE WHEAT BREAD: A handful of unsalted peanuts or a couple tablespoons of all-natural peanut butter can provide a big energy boost. In a study conducted at Pennsylvania State University, children whose diets included moderate amounts of peanuts had higher intakes of protein, fiber, vitamin A, vitamin E, and other vital nutrients than those who did not. Energy intake was significantly higher. And although they consumed more fat, peanuts contain healthy, monounsaturated fat, so mean body mass index was lower for peanut-eaters than non-peanut eaters.

Not That!
FAST FOOD: Kids who eat out at restaurants more than four times per week have higher blood pressure, lower HDL levels, and higher intake of starch, sugar, sodium, fat, and cholesterol than those who eat at home, according to the American Heart Association. What's more, frequent fast-food eaters drink twice as much soda and are significantly less physically active than their peers.

Eat This, Not That!

HELP YOUR KIDS MAKE THE RIGHT DECISION EVERY TIME

McDonald's

Eat This

Happy Meal®

Chicken McNuggets® (4 pc), Apple Dippers with low-fat caramel dip, and 1% Low Fat Milk Jug (8 fl oz)

375 calories 13 g fat (3.5 g saturated) 610 mg sodium

Not That!

Happy Meal®

Cheeseburger, Apple Dippers with low-fat caramel dip, and 1% Low Fat Chocolate Milk Jug (8 fl oz)

575 calories 16 g fat (8 g saturated) 935 mg sodium

Burger King

Eat This

Chicken Tenders®

(4 piece) with strawberry applesauce and 1% milk

370 calories 12.5 g fat (2.5 g saturated) 610 mg sodium

Not That!

Cheeseburger

with small fries and orange juice

700 calories 29 g fat (10 g saturated) 1,180 mg sodium

Wendy's

Eat This

Ham & Cheese Sandwich Kids' Meal

200 calories 5 g fat (2.5 g saturated) 810 mg sodium

Not That!

Cheeseburger Kids' Meal

260 calories 11 g fat (5 g saturated) 710 mg sodium

Taco Bell

Eat This

Spicy Chicken Soft Taco

170 calories 6 g fat (2 g saturated) 580 mg sodium

Not That!

Cheesy Fiesta Potatoes

290 calories 17 g fat (4 g saturated) 830 mg sodium

Chili's

Eat This

Pepper Pals® Little Mouth Burger

280 calories   15 g fat (5 g saturated)
300 mg sodium

Not That!

Pepper Pals® Crispy Honey Chipotle Crispers (3 crispers)

770 calories   41 g fat (8 g saturated)
1,870 mg sodium

Subway

Eat This

Ham Mini Sub

180 calories   3 g fat (1 g saturated)
710 mg sodium

Not That!

Tuna Mini Sub

320 calories   18 g fat (4.5 g saturated)
690 mg sodium

Denny's

Eat This

Kid's D-Zone Smiley-Alien Hotcakes

230 calories   3 g fat (.5 g saturated)
710 mg sodium

Not That!

Kid's D-Zone Junior Grand Slam®

400 calories   21 g fat (7 g saturated)
900 mg sodium

Panera

Eat This

Panera Kids Grilled Cheese sandwich

290 calories   11 g fat (6 g saturated)
890 mg sodium

Not That!

Panera Kids Smoked Ham deli sandwich

360 calories   14 g fat (7 g saturated)
1,490 mg sodium

Romano's Macaroni Grill

Eat This

Kid's Spaghetti & Meatballs with Tomato Sauce

500 calories   20 g fat (8 g saturated)
1,520 mg sodium

Not That!

Kid's Double Macaroni 'n' Cheese

1,210 calories   62 g fat (40 g saturated)
3,450 mg sodium

Index

Boldface page references indicate photographs.
<u>Underscored</u> references indicate boxed text, graphs, or tables.

Lose Your Gut
& Stay Healthy

with The Abs Diet Online

If you loved Eat This, Not That, wait until you try the revolutionary weight loss plan from the editor-in-chief of Men's Health.

- Personalized nutrition plans with plenty of real-food options
- Flexible, customized workout programs designed to fit your schedule, not dictate it
- Convenient, confidential 24/7 access anywhere you can get online
- Based on the best-selling book, The Abs Diet

SIGN UP TODAY FOR YOUR 30-DAY FREE TRIAL

the AbsDiet®online

absdietonline.com/offer

200921201

Check out the *New York Times* best-selling Abs Diet series
also available from David Zinczenko

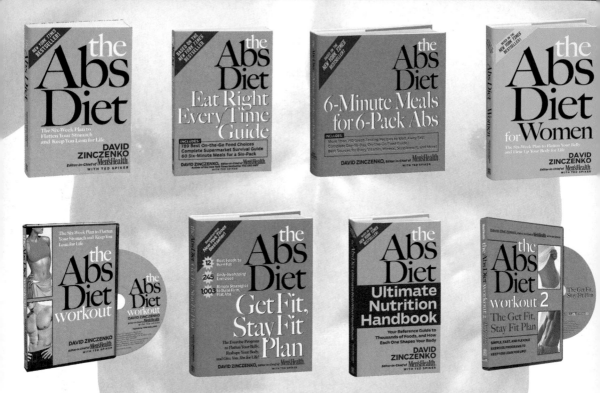

The Abs Diet series, by *Men's Health* editor-in-chief David Zinczenko, has helped hundreds of thousands of people lose pounds quickly and dramatically reshape their bodies. In just 6 weeks, you too can achieve a flatter stomach and better shape—and learn how to stay lean and healthy for life.

AVAILABLE WHEREVER BOOKS AND DVDS ARE SOLD OR VISIT ABSDIET.COM

For more of our products visit www.rodalestore.com or call (800) 848-4735

RODALE
LIVE YOUR WHOLE LIFE